Understanding Depression

Understanding Depression

by

PAUL R. ROBBINS

McFarland & Company, Inc., Publishers
Jefferson, North Carolina, and London

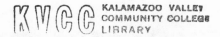

MAR 1 6 1995

British Library Cataloguing-in-Publication data are available

Library of Congress Cataloguing-in-Publication Data

Robbins, Paul R. (Paul Richard)
    Understanding depression / by Paul R. Robbins.
    p. cm.
    Includes bibliographical references and index.
    ISBN 0-89950-878-2 (lib. bdg. : 50# alk. paper) ∞
    1. Depression, Mental—Popular works. I. Title.
RC537.R58 1993
616.85′27—dc20   92-56685
                                                         CIP

Manufactured in the United States of America

McFarland & Company, Inc., Publishers
  Box 611, Jefferson, North Carolina 28640

To the memory of Edith Robbins

Acknowledgments

Grateful acknowledgment is made to the following for permission to reprint excerpts from their copyrighted materials. Plenum Publishing Corporation for S. D. Hollon and P. C. Kendall, Cognitive self-statements in depression: Development of an automatic thoughts questionnaire, *Cognitive Therapy and Research*, 4 (1980): 383–95 and J. D. Safran, M. Vallis, Z. V. Segal, and B. F. Shaw, Assessment of core cognitive processes in cognitive therapy, *Cognitive Therapy and Research* 10 (1986): 509–26. Clinical Psychology Publishing Co., Inc., Brandon, VT 05733 for P. R. Robbins, and J. F. Nugent, III, Perceived consequences of addiction: A comparison between alcoholics and heroin-addicted patients, *Journal of Clinical Psychology* 31 (1975): 367–69. *Psychiatry* for H. A. Meyersburg, S. L. Ablon, and J. Kotin, A reverberating psychic mechanism in the depressive processes, *Psychiatry*, 37 (1974): 372–86. Farrar, Straus and Giroux, Inc., for J. Anouilh, *The Restless Heart*, in *Jean Anouilh Five Plays*, volume 2. Copyright 1959 by Hill and Wang, Inc.

Table of Contents

Introduction

Most people "get depressed" now and then. It's a sad feeling, being in the dumps. The feeling is usually transient, vanishing in hours or days, like the proverbial dark clouds that give way to sunshine. We think of such short-lived depressed states as *depressed moods*, not to be confused with the often chronic, severe problem called *clinical depression*.

Transient depressed moods may be as common as the cold. My colleague Roland Tanck and I carried out a series of studies on college students in which we asked the students to fill out a special type of diary before they went to bed for a period of ten nights. The diary included the question "Did you feel depressed today?" There were very few students who did not answer the question yes at some time during the ten-day period, and many students said yes repeatedly.

Going to college is not easy. There are major adjustments that must be made in being away from home. Problems in relationships develop with frequent disappointments. Term papers are due and examinations generate a great deal of stress. One might expect to observe depressed moods in students, and one finds them in abundance. Still, most of the students do not stay depressed. They get over romantic disappointments, pass their exams, and continue to study and go about their daily lives. Brief periods of depressed mood give way to more pleasant moods. Good times are often right around the corner.

In clinical depression there is a sharp contrast. Often, the clinically depressed person doesn't see a corner. He or she may not even see that there is a possibility of a corner. Clinical depression is something like being in a black hole. The person feels trapped and the future may appear hopeless.

This perception of hopelessness is often accompanied by deep feelings of sadness, loss of interest in what had previously made life meaningful and sometimes thoughts of suicide. The depressed person often has slowed reactions, trouble concentrating and remembering, difficulty in sleeping and sometimes a marked weight loss. When such problems persist over time, we are talking about an emotional illness that merits careful evaluation and appropriate therapy. I shall have much to say about the options for treatment that are available and I hope the discussion will prove useful if seeking professional help is under consideration.

Between the occasional blue moods of everyday life and a severe clinical depression, there are millions of people who experience periods of mild to moderate depressed mood. They may experience some of the same symptoms of the clinically depressed person, such as difficulties in sleeping and feelings of sadness. Such people enjoy life much less than they would like. At times, their daily routine seems like drudgery, but they continue to function, going to school, working and taking care of their children. The depressed state diminishes the quality of life, but life goes on.

There is a lot that such depressed people can do to create a happier, more rewarding life for themselves. In this book I shall present some ideas and information that I hope will assist them in moving toward this goal. However, the book is not intended as a substitute for therapy if that is what is needed. I believe that this book will also be helpful to those who know or live with people who are prone to depression. The information that shall be presented may help these people better understand what is happening to their friend or loved one.

To fulfill these objectives, I shall present in the first chapters of the book a picture of what is currently known about depressed moods and depression. In the final chapters I shall offer some ideas about how to prevent depressed moods and how to cope with these moods when they occur.

1. Depressed Mood and Depression

Your mood colors the way you perceive your environment, the people about you and yourself. If you are in a happy mood, you tend to look at others and yourself through rose-colored glasses. Everything seems right with the world. There is, indeed, some truth in the feeling that when you're happy, the whole world is happy, too. People may not be happy in reality but if you're happy, it may not matter that much.

When you are feeling in a sad mood, you tend to look at things with a negative perspective. Gone are the rose-colored glasses. Now you are wearing very dark ones. And this overflow of bleak mood can affect the way you look at yourself.

An interesting experiment demonstrates how mood may influence judgment. Before describing the experiment, I should state that researchers have developed techniques that can be used to alter the mood of normal subjects.

One of these mood induction techniques is hypnosis. Another comparatively simple technique that has been widely used is to ask the subject to read a set of standardized phrases that are sad in content.[1] An example would be, "The way I feel now, the future looks boring and hopeless." It has been repeatedly demonstrated that when people read these phrases and *feel the mood* as they do so—they become more depressed. In contrast, reading happy phrases tends to elevate mood. Mood can be that sensitive to change!

The experiment I am going to describe was carried out by Joseph Forgas and his colleagues. For the experiment, the subjects were first interviewed for a while on a variety of topics. These interviews were

---

[1] *The technique was developed by E. Velten (1986).*

1

videotaped with the subjects' consent. On the following day, the subjects were given a mood induction technique to make them feel either happier or sadder about themselves. The subjects were then asked to make judgments about their own videotapes. The subjects in the positive mood judged their performance as competent, confident and socially skilled. The subjects who had been put in a negative mood saw their previous performances as incompetent, clumsy and unskilled. Objective judges did not see any difference in the two sets of interviews. It was all in the minds of the subjects.

If depressed mood can make you think more negatively, it is equally true that negative thoughts can depress your mood. Drawing on this observation, Aaron T. Beck has developed one of the most influential theories about the cause of depression, as well as an effective form of therapy, called *cognitive therapy*. When mood and thinking patterns are negative, you may also see changes in behavior, such as slowed reactions and a loss of interest in your usual activities. Moreover, there may be changes in the way you feel physically. A person may have a variety of physical complaints and not sleep or eat as well as before. Instead of a simple depressed mood, what we now have is a more complex situation — a mixture of symptoms. This group of symptoms is called depression.

The clinical description and understanding of depression has become refined in recent years, but the notion that people can become saddened and immobilized goes back a long way. Hippocrates and Aretaeus, physicians of ancient Greece, wrote about people who suffered from a form of depressive illness. The Greeks used the word *melancholia* to describe depression, naming the condition after one of the hypothetical bodily humors they believed influenced mood.[2] In later centuries, the belief existed that depression was the work of the devil.

The world's literature has its share of characters who appear depressed. One finds depressed people in literary works ranging from the tales of "A Thousand and One Nights" to the writings of the German poet and dramatist Johann Wolfgang von Goethe.[3] Remember the despondent figure of King Lear in Shakespeare or the guilt-ridden Lady Macbeth?

---

[2]*Four fluids (cardinal humors) were thought to influence one's health: blood, phlegm, choler, and melancholy (black bile).*
[3]*See Goethe (1774), p. 1.*

Among historical figures, Abraham Lincoln was described as a melancholy man. He wrote to his law partner, John Stuart, "I am now the most miserable man living. If what I feel were equally distributed to the whole human family, there would not be one cheerful face on earth. Whether I shall ever be better, I cannot tell: I awfully forebode I shall not. To remain as I am is impossible. I must die or be better . . . ."[4] Composers Robert Schumann, Hector Berlioz and George Frideric Handel, novelist Virginia Woolf and poets Lord Byron and Robert Lowell were among the creative talents who suffered from depression.

The presence of depression in such famous people has led to speculation on whether there is an association between depressive disorders and creativity. A study was conducted of over one thousand persons selected from the *British Dictionary of National Biography*. The sample included people in the sciences, arts and politics. About one out of twelve persons in the sample were said to have melancholia, a figure that is not strikingly high.[5] However, other studies suggest that artists and writers might be particularly vulnerable to depression. In one study it was reported that 38 percent of a sample of artists and writers had been treated for depressive illness.[6]

While the concept of depression has its roots in early times, the attempt to clearly define it as a clinical disorder had to await the development of psychiatry in the nineteenth century. The description and classification of mental and emotional disorders gained great impetus during the latter half of the nineteenth century, much of it resulting from the pioneering efforts of German psychiatrist Emil Kraepelin. In eight editions of his *Textbook of Psychiatry*, he distinguished between different types of mental illness, using such terms as manic-depressive disorder, which remain part of psychiatric language today.

The attempts to describe and classify what appeared to be different types or shadings of depression have continued since Kraepelin's time. Various descriptive terms have entered the psychiatric literature, proving more-or-less useful, including *involutional melancholia, endogeneous depression, reactive depression, neurotic depression,* and *dysthymic disorder.* Dysthymic disorder may be the least familiar of these names, but is a term in current favor that refers to depression which is

---

[4]*See Folkenberg (1983), p. 1.*
[5]*See Ellis (1926).*
[6]*DeAngelis (1989), p. 24. These data were obtained by Kay R. Jamison.*

typically not severe but is long lasting, the type of problem that may linger for years. Despite this formidable sounding list of diagnostic categories, the problem of meaningfully distinguishing between varieties of depressive problems is not fully settled. The American Psychiatric Association, through its task forces and committees, has been wrestling with the problem. The association's current thinking is embodied in its *Diagnostic and Statistical Manual of Mental Disorders.*[7] While there is some uncertainty concerning the subtypings of depression, there is general agreement about the typical symptoms of depression. I shall now describe these symptoms.

Symptoms of Depression

I have briefly alluded to some of the symptoms that characterize depression. I will now take a more detailed look at them. One of the clearest signs is mood. A sad, blue mood that persists is usually a dead giveaway that something is wrong. Sadness is sometimes visible in facial expressions. Depressed people may look glum and downcast. Using the electromyograph to measure activity of the muscles, one can study the facial muscles of depressed people. For example, electrodes can be placed near the eyes to monitor the corrugator muscles, which pull the eyebrows down. EMG readings for these muscles tend to be higher in depressed people and may be even higher when depressed people think unhappy thoughts.

There are times in life when sadness is a normal, expected response to unhappy or tragic events. Bereavement is such a time and we expect a period of grief and mourning as part of a psychological healing process. But protracted sadness under any circumstances is something to be concerned about.

A second sign that a person is depressed is a loss of interest and pleasure in his or her usual activities and pursuits. The person may simply go through the motions or even stop the activities altogether. An example would be Arlene, once an enthusiastic gardener, interested in cooking and entertaining, active in her church. Her enthusiasm for all of these activities has dwindled. When her friends asked her about this,

---

[7]*This important reference has gone through several revisions. The current edition is known as DSM III-R. A fourth edition is now in preparation.*

she replied, "I don't care anymore." What was important and fulfilling in her life had lost its meaning.

Another sign of depression is excessive self-reproach. Therapists who have worked with depressed patients have observed that many depressed patients are overly self-critical. Freud described depressed patients in the following way: "The patient represents his ego to us as worthless, incapable of any effort, and morally despicable; he reproaches himself, villifies himself and expects to be cast out and chastised."[8] Depressed people may feel responsible for events they really have no control over. They are often overly concerned with their own faults, shortcomings and failings. The message may boil down to "I'm no good." The flip side of this conclusion is often "I deserve to be punished."

Many depressed people carry with them a large burden of guilt, a painful feeling that they have violated the standards of what is right and wrong, what is acceptable and unacceptable. These standards have strong emotional roots in childhood learning experiences and particularly in the moral teachings of parents. To feel you have violated these expectations can be a wrenching experience.

In addition to the substantial clinical observation that feelings of self-reproach and guilt are often part of a depressive picture,[9] there is some experimental evidence that activating guilt may deepen the depressed mood, and that this may happen on an unconscious level. The process may take place without any awareness.

The experimental procedure used in these studies is interesting, though controversial, as it utilized the not-fully-understood technique of subliminal perception. Depressed subjects viewed short sentences or phrases at such rapid speeds of exposure that they were unable to make out what they were looking at. What the subjects saw was something like a flash or a blur. When researchers used phrases like "leaving Mom is wrong" or "I have been bad," the subject's mood after the experiment became more depressed. The effect was clearest in subjects who seemed more guilt-prone on psychological testing.[10]

---

[8]*Freud (1959), p. 155.*

[9]*The empirical studies that have examined guilt in depressed patients seem to confirm the clinical picture. Robin Jarrett and Jan Weissenburger, for example, found that depressed patients reported higher levels of guilt than control subjects in a variety of situations: doing unintentional harm, failure of self-control, disregard for relationships, expression of anger, failure to meet need and violation of principles. Jarrett & Weissenburger (1990).*

[10]*See Dauber (1984) and the doctoral thesis of Schmidt (1981).*

Thoughts of suicide are another sign of depression. Sometimes these thoughts are expressed in verbal statements that are direct and unmistakable. Sometimes the idea of suicide is expressed obliquely and not easily recognizable. The possibility of suicide in depression must be taken very seriously. Estimates are that the lifetime risk of suicide in persons with serious depression runs on the order of 15 percent while it is only about 1 percent for the general population.[11]

Trouble in sleeping is another possible indication of depression. Obviously, not everybody who has trouble sleeping is depressed, but so many people who are depressed have difficulty sleeping that this problem is often a tell-tale sign. Sometimes the problem is what is called *sleep onset insomnia*. The person goes to bed at night and can't fall asleep. Instead of lapsing into sleep, the person may begin to rethink and replay the events of the day or troubling unresolved problems. As the person lies in bed, these thoughts may repeat themselves over and over, something like a phonograph record that is stuck in a groove. When we ask a depressed patient what he or she was thinking about while struggling to sleep, we often gain a pretty good encapsulation of what some of the person's major problems are.

Many depressed patients appear to have slowed reactions. This tendency might include both slowness in sizing up a situation and in responding. While it is difficult to separate these two components of reaction in real life, efforts have been made to do so in laboratory experiments. Research has shown that compared to normal controls, depressed patients are slower in making physical reactions.[12]

When people are extremely depressed, their body movements may have a uniform, monotonous, limited character. Picture in your mind the graceful movements of a dancer, then imagine what the opposite of that might be like. In a metaphorical sense, it is as if the restriction in the patients' movements mirror the restriction in their current lives. When depressed patients begin to improve, constricted body motion begins to become more mobile, complex and dynamic.

Chronic fatigue is yet another sign of possible depression. While all of us get tired at times, depressed people often feel tired and lethargic. To get out of bed in the morning may seem like a tremendous task. For some depressed people, the day seems to drag like a clock going in slow

[11]*Gallagher (1986), p. 4.*
[12]*See Cornell et al. (1984).*

motion and the person may feel about as energetic as the clock. When a person reports chronic fatigue and there is no clear physiological basis for it, one must be alert to the possibility of an underlying depression.

The eating disorders *anorexia* and *bulimia* are now in the public consciousness, thanks to a spate of books and magazine articles. These articles have heightened our awareness of the impact of emotional problems on the way we approach and consume food. Changes in eating habits, which are reflected in large weight gains or losses, may also be an indicator of depression. Obviously, if a person is clearly overweight and trying to lose weight, this benchmark for depression should not apply.

Returning to bulimia for a moment, it is interesting that many people with this problem have experienced depression during their lives. The prevalence of depression in bulimics is far above what one finds in the general population. It could be that discontent with one's self plays a role in both the purgative behavior and depressed feelings one finds in many bulimics.

Diminished ability to concentrate and remember things is also a possible sign of depression. Patients will often complain of this problem in their jobs or school work. The problem is real enough: a number of experimental studies show that people who are depressed may not remember verbal materials as well as people who are not depressed. In a paper reviewing this research, Mark Johnson and Peter Magaro stated, "Given the frequent complaints of memory impairment reported by depressed patients, a number of investigators have attempted to verify this phenomena experimentally. The majority of these investigations have examined memory processes in depressed inpatient samples. Most have demonstrated some memory impairments when depressed patients are compared with normal nonpsychiatric control groups."[13] Generally speaking, the more severe the depression is, the greater the problems with memory. When the depression begins to clear up, memory tends to improve.

One possible explanation for the difficulties in memory experienced by many people who are depressed is that they are often very preoccupied with their own problems. This self-focusing may interfere with their ability to concentrate on the external world and communications coming from others. It is hard to remember things when it is a problem paying attention to what is going on about you.

[13]*Johnson & Magaro (1987), p. 29.*

When a person has been feeling in a depressed mood—even in a mild one—she or he will often report more physical complaints. As an illustration of this pattern, consider some research Roland Tanck and I carried out using our student diaries.

We asked the students whether they were feeling depressed during the day. We also asked them whether they had been experiencing any physical symptoms during the day. To assist the students in recording these symptoms, we provided a list of physical complaints such as headaches, nausea, dizziness, weakness and diarrhea, and asked the students to check off any of the complaints they had experienced. The students who reported feeling higher levels of depressed mood reported more physical complaints.

Depressed mood has a relation with physical symptoms. It is not, however, easy to establish what is cause and what is effect. It is possible that the depressed mood may cause physical problems. However, it is also possible that a person may react to physical problems by becoming depressed.

Measuring Depression

These, then, are some of the typical symptoms of depression. How do we measure depression as a practical matter? How do we say that this person has a mild depression or that person has a more serious problem? The standard used for diagnosing a person as depressed is a clinical interview conducted by trained psychiatrists or psychologists using a set of benchmark criteria similar to the symptoms we have described. A good deal of research, however, has demonstrated that you can get a reasonably good estimate of what the clinicians would find in their interviews by using questionnaires in which people report their own symptoms. One of the most widely used of these self-report measures is a 21-item inventory developed by Aaron Beck of the University of Pennsylvania.[14] Another inventory used in community studies on depression was developed by the National Institutes of Health's Center for Epidemiological Studies.[15]

---

[14]*The Beck Depression Inventory (BDI) has been used extensively in research with both clinically depressed and nondepressed subjects. See Beck et al. (1961).*
[15]*See Radloff (1977).*

These inventories are easy to administer and score and are very convenient to use in carrying out research on depression. One drawback of these inventories is that they have a tendency to give an inflated picture of the prevalence of depression. Research suggests that many people who would be considered depressed on the basis of a self-report questionnaire would not be evaluated as depressed in a clinical interview.

While I will not reproduce any of the published inventories, I would like to give you an idea of the types of questions that are used in self-report measures of depression. Following are some questions that are similar to those used in depression inventories:

1. Have you experienced extended periods of sadness during the past few weeks?
2. Have you been having problems sleeping?
3. Has your appetite been poor lately?
4. Have you been more withdrawn from people in recent weeks?
5. Have you felt tired a lot of the time?
6. Have you noticed that you have little enthusiasm about doing things?
7. Have you been down on yourself lately?
8. Do you find that you are getting much less satisfaction from your usual activities than you used to?
9. Have you recently been troubled by feelings of guilt?
10. Do you often feel like crying?
11. Have you been experiencing feelings of deep pessimism?
12. Have you recently been troubled by physical symptoms such as headaches, nausea, or dizziness?
13. Have you noticed a decline in your desire for having a sexual experience?
14. Have you been feeling that you are very much alone in life?
15. Have you noticed you have had difficulty lately in concentrating on your work?
16. Do you find yourself sluggish in your reactions?
17. Do you have feelings that nothing in life seems worthwhile?
18. Have you been feeling overwhelmed by the problems you have been facing in life?
19. Have you been thinking that you are a failure in life?
20. Have people been telling you that you seem depressed?

The sample of preceding questions is a collection of items, *not a psychological test*. We would have to show by research that a score based on the responses to such items is a reliable and valid measure before we could interpret the results with any precision. Having said this, if you answered the questions and found that you had only a few "yes" answers, it seems unlikely that you would have a serious depressive problem. On the other hand, if you answered most of the questions yes, you might want to consider consulting a mental health professional to discuss the things that are bothering you.

As we have indicated, most of us experience times in which our mood is sad or blue and we may experience some of the symptoms of depression. What makes these symptoms more serious or less serious is how *intense* they are and how *long* they persist. Take mood for example. You can feel a little blue or you can feel just terrible. It is the latter condition you worry about. There is no absolute rule of thumb for how long depressed feelings persist before you should begin to feel concerned, but certainly a couple of weeks of intense symptoms is more than enough time to recognize that you ought to do something about it. The American Psychiatric Association's *Diagnostic and Statistical Manual* suggests that two weeks of intense symptoms is enough to classify what is happening as a major depressive episode.

While we are discussing measurement, let's consider the measurement of mood. In contrast to the measurement of depressed states — which may require use of a variety of questions to explore a number of different symptoms such as sleep and appetite disturbances — the measurement of mood seems straightforward. We are able to assess a person's mood in surprisingly easy ways. One such technique is to use the Adjective Check List.

Let's say a researcher is trying to find out what your mood is like at this moment. To do this, he or she might ask you to respond with a list of words that describe various moods. The list will have been refined with the aid of statistical procedures so that the researcher can derive scores to represent the intensity of different moods, such as anger, anxiety or depression. To give you an idea how these techniques work, we have drawn up a list of words that are similar to those used in standardized adjective check lists. As was true for our questions about depression, this is not a psychological test, simply a way of showing how researchers study mood.

If you are interested, try responding to the list of words using the following procedure. Look at each word in the list in turn. If you don't feel in the mood described at all, check the box on the left. If you feel a little bit in the mood described, check the box in the center. If you definitely feel that way, check the box on the right.

	Not at All	A Little Bit	Definitely
Affectionate	☐	☑	☑
Alert	☐	☐	☑
Angry	☐	☐	☑
Anxious	☐	☐	☑
Blue	☐	☑	☐
Cheerful	☐	☑	☐
Contemplative	☐	☑	☐
Dejected	☐	☑	☐
Distraught	☐	☑	☐
Downhearted	☐	☑	☐
Energetic	☑	☐	☐
Fearful	☐	☐	☑
Friendly	☐	☐	☑
Glad	☐	☑	☐
Gloomy	☐	☑	☐
Happy	☐	☑	☐
Irritable	☐	☑	☐
Jittery	☐	☑	☐
Joyful	☐	☑	☐
Kindly	☐	☑	☐
Lethargic	☐	☑	☐
Merry	☐	☑	☐
Optimistic	☐	☐	☑
Pessimistic	☐	☐	☑
Pleasant	☐	☑	☐
Relaxed	☐	☑	☐
Restful	☐	☑	☐
Sad	☐	☑	☐
Sociable	☐	☑	☐
Suspicious	☐	☐	☑
Thoughtful	☐	☑	☐
Tired	☐	☐	☑
Worried	☐	☐	☑

Look at the words for which you checked "Definitely." What kinds of moods do these words suggest? Look at the words you checked "Not at All." What kinds of moods do these words suggest? Do you see any patterns? Now, take a closer look at the words *Blue, Dejected, Distraught, Downhearted, Gloomy, Pessimistic* and *Sad.* If you checked "Definitely" for several of these words, chances are that your mood at the moment is depressed. Mood changes: If you check this list again tomorrow, you might find a different pattern. When depressed mood persists, however, there is a problem.

Mood Swings

It would be a very rare person indeed whose moods are constant. Some of us have moods like shifting winds. We react to changes in body chemistry, to events in our environment and to our thought processes — conscious, and in the psychoanalytic view, unconscious as well. As we have indicated, it is possible to induce a depressed mood by simply reading and trying "to feel" a list of depressive phrases.

If you think about it you can probably recall books that you have read or movies you have seen that left you feeling depressed. Try listening to the last movement of Tchaikovsky's *Pathétique* Symphony (no. 6). It can be a real downer.

The other side of this process is mood elevation. Try thinking of people, parties, music, vacations, books, sporting events — good times that have elevated your mood, producing a sense of well being.

We mentioned that body chemistry can influence mood. A good example of this is the premenstrual syndrome (PMS) experienced by many women. These women may feel depressed, anxious and irritable during the premenstrual phase of the menstrual cycle. It is a little difficult to estimate how many women experience *premenstrual depression* because many women who have this problem also experience intermittent depression at other times during the month. However, there are studies which suggest that about 40 percent of the women who report PMS depression experience an increase in depressed mood *only* in the premenstrual period and return to a normal mood after menstruation ceases.[16]

What kind of variation in mood do you experience during a day?

---

[16]*See McMillan & Pihl (1987).*

Are you more likely to be bursting with enthusiasm during the day and dropping off as the day ends? Or are you a grumbler in the morning and a free spirit in the evening? Are you a night person?

Roland Tanck and I were interested in the problem of mood swings within the day and used our diaries to obtain some information from college students. The results might surprise you. If you feel brighter during the day and your mood deteriorates somewhat as evening falls, you are not alone.

In reflecting upon their day's experiences, most of the students reported that typically the downside of mood was in the evening. The students felt best during various times of the day, but by evening, the day's activities seem to have taken a toll on them and their mood deteriorated. A night's sleep seemed to clear things up and they were ready to go in the morning.

We found fewer instances of the reverse pattern, of "night people"—students who felt more depressed in the morning and peaked in the evening.

Some students in our sample reported having periods of depressed mood that persisted right through the day with little evidence of mood swing. It was these students with stretches of rather constant depressed mood who were more likely to report the typical symptoms of depression such as a plethora of physical complaints.

Mood Swings in Clinical Depression

Many years ago I remember a young man who came to see me in the middle of winter. He told me how life seemed so "draggy" in the winter, but how he felt so much better in the summer when he played tennis and softball. I thought part of the problem might be the recent holiday season and we talked about the feelings he experienced in being alone and away from home during Christmas. Still, this did not seem to be the crux of the problem. During therapy he alluded several times to the feeling that everything seemed so dark and dreary in the winter. I suggested that he try lighting up his apartment with bright lights and see if that might help. I don't know whether he thought going to a therapist who offered such simple-minded advice was a poor investment, but he ceased coming soon afterwards.

Some years later, I began to read of a new concept called *seasonal affective disorder.* Patients report they feel OK in the sunlit days of summer but feel terrible during the dark days of winter. Dr. Norman Rosenthal has been largely responsible for developing the idea. Among the therapies that seem effective in treating this mid-winter case of the blahs are very bright lights. Interestingly, artificial light therapy seems to work best when it is carried out in the morning. Perhaps it mimics the pleasant sensation of awakening on a bright summer day. In any event, I was delighted to learn that my off-the-cuff suggestion to a patient was not idiotic after all.

There have been reports that seasonal depression may work the other way as well—feeling OK in the winter and depressed in the summer. This seems somewhat harder to explain than its counterpart. A case of this atypical pattern of seasonal depression was described by Thomas Wehr and his colleagues:

> Ms. A, a 66-year-old married retired secretary, had had recurrent summer depressions, beginning in March–April and ending in August–October, for at least 15 years. When depressed, she was indecisive, had negative thoughts, and scarcely spoke. She had frequent crying spells and suicidal thoughts. Because of lethargy, lack of motivation, and difficulty concentrating, she engaged in no activity voluntarily and tried to sleep as much as possible. In the fall and winter she was energetic and outgoing. She required less sleep, was talkative and had racing thoughts.
>
> Her clinical state appeared to be influenced by changes in climate and weather. Her depressions began earlier than usual during spring vacations in Florida, and remissions occurred during midsummer vacations in New England. . . . We observed a temporary remission when an unusual cold front reduced the temperature to 39°F in June. Furthermore, she appeared to improve after an experimental cold treatment, as just described.[17]

Researchers have been studying people reporting seasonal depression, comparing them with people whose depression is not seasonal. One interesting observation is that the seasonal depressives do not have difficulties in getting enough sleep. They often sleep too much. In addition, they may have very good appetites—and often have a tendency to crave carbohydrates. The speculation is that carbohydrate binging may have something to do with biochemical deficiencies in the neurotransmitter serotonin. I shall have more to say about the role of the neurotransmitters in depression in later chapters.

[17]*Wehr et al. (1987), p. 1603.*

Bipolar Depression

The clinical disorder of *bipolar depression* is characterized by pronounced shifts in mood. The disorder was recognized in the mid nineteenth century by a physician named J. P. Falret, who published descriptions of manic excitement and depression and used the term *circular insanity* to describe the phenomenon. This legalistic and pejorative term never received much currency and was replaced by the diagnostic labels of *manic depressive disorder* and *bipolar disorder,* which have essentially the same meanings. The key elements in bipolar disorder are dramatic swings in mood. At times the patient may be very depressed, reporting many of the symptoms in our earlier description of clinical depression. However, at other times, the patient will be in a hyperelated state, which has been termed *mania* or *hypomania,* depending on severity. The patient may engage in a whirlwind of activities, thoughts firing rapidly from one idea to the next and speech difficult to interpret. The need for sleep seems to vanish. Self-esteem becomes inflated. Prudence may disappear and the patient may do some very rash things.

In a manic state the patient may make all kinds of plans, look up old friends—sometimes calling them in the middle of the night—go on buying sprees, even drive recklessly. This state of euphoric mood and hyperexcitement seems like it is 180 degree away from the patient's depressed state. Hence the term bipolar disorder.

People who have this problem go through cycles with manic episodes, depressive episodes and normal periods. A revealing study carried out by Richard Depue and his colleagues tell us a good deal about the behavior of people with bipolar depressive problems. The subjects in the study had bipolar problems but were not at that time impaired enough to require hospitalization. They reported increased and decreased energy patterns, uneven patterns of productivity, mental confusion, high and low sociability patterns, high and low interest patterns, increased and decreased sleep patterns, and highs and lows in sexual interest.

Depue reported that typically depressed episodes lasted from three to six days. The duration of manic episodes was about the same—two to six days. About two-thirds of his subjects had between two and six depressed episodes per year with about the same numbers holding for manic episodes. The impression one gets from these statistics is that the outbreaks of bipolar symptoms were fairly frequent, but time limited. For

Depue's sample of people whose problems were not serious enough to require hospitalization, the episodes seemed to run their course.

The researchers describe a case that illuminates some of the clinical features of bipolar disorder. The subject, Miss S, is an 18-year-old college student. The researchers first describe some of the behaviors of her hypomanic phase. Following are some excerpts:

> *Mood.* Feeling clearly higher or happier than is usually the case, "as if I have a different personality, I feel hyper, and I fool around a great deal, laughing and joking all the time." Other people notice the change in mood and comment to her about it.
>
> *Energy and need for excitement.* She has greatly increased energy that "goes with the high feelings." People comment on this, usually saying that she "ought to slow down" or that she is "wearing them out." She participates in many more sports activities, goes more places than usual ("to see people, stores, bars, anywhere"), and does other activities that she might not ordinarily do. During these active times she can get so excited that she is unable to sit still, and she jumps from one activity to another.
>
> She reports an intense need for excitement, and begins new activities with lots of enthusiasm and then quickly loses interest in them. For instance, in one recent phase, she started skiing lessons, two new embroidery works, needlepoint lessons, learning a new complicated card game, and she joined a women's group, but dropped all of them at the end of her 2-week hypomanic period. . . .
>
> *Thoughts, speech and distractibility.* During these phases her thoughts race so fast that she "can say about one half of a thought and then it is gone." Also, her attention jumps rapidly from one thought to another so that she loses her "train of thought totally." At these times, she talks very fast, and stumbles over words, and others complain that they cannot hold a conversation with her. . . .
>
> *Irresponsible behavior.* She spends money she cannot afford or other people's money. . . . [S]he is sexually active with new male friends, which leads to trouble with her steady boyfriend; she gets into a lot of verbal, and sometimes physical, fights; she frequents bars more and drinks more when she goes to bars; she drives recklessly (goes through red lights and stop signs) and faster than usual (more than 10 miles over the speed limit, whereas this is not usual for her).

The authors then describe the behaviors of her depressive phases.

> *Mood.* Both depression and irritability, but mainly the former. Others always tell her she looks sad or depressed during "lows," and the feeling is described as "painful." Nonverbal cues of depression are apparently evident in facial expression, since others always comment on her depression, and she has frequent crying spells, without understanding why, and has an almost constant urge to cry. . . .

Energy and motor activity. During "lows" she feels very tired and worn out. She does not do school work ("couldn't if I tried"). She could manage to go out, but she "wouldn't go out on my own initiative." She reports that she is "slowed down" and that "moving is more difficult."

Concentration. Her concentration is poor; it is "difficult or impossible to read."

Somatic complaints. Her somatic complaints are frequent during "lows" (headaches, blurred vision, constipation; vacillates between feeling too hot and too cold). . . .

Cognitions. She reports a range of negative cognitions, including indecision over small matters, pessimism about present and future, being a burden to her family, that she would be better off dead. . . .

Miss S had been experiencing hypomanic and depressive periods since her first year of junior high school. It was reported that she might experience four phases in a year, each of which would last for at least two continuous weeks.[18]

In some bipolar patients, we encounter alterations in mood that occur much more frequently than was the case for Miss S. These patients seem to be constantly shifting from one mood extremity to the other, a pattern called *rapid cycling of mood.* In some patients, rapid cycling may take place in 48 hours. Imagine what confusion such changes can generate. Rapid cycling may be related to endocrine disturbances and has also been reported as a rare effect of taking certain antidepressant medications.

Infrequently, one sees cases reported of rapid cycling in unipolar depression—from normal mood to depressed and back again—all happening very regularly and quickly. Sidney Zisook reported a case, Mrs. L, who experienced states of normalcy and depression alternating every other day. On one day she felt fine, energetic and cheerful. On the next day she had many of the classic symptoms of depression—her energy, appetite and ability to enjoy life were all diminished. The alterations in mood were as regular as clockwork. Neither Mrs. L nor her physicians understood the nature of her problem; for too long she was written off as a chronic complainer.[19]

Miss S and Mrs. L are people who have experienced perplexing mood swings that have troubled and complicated their lives. As we shall

---

[18]*Depue et al. (1981), pp. 436–37.*

[19]*For an analysis of mood fluctuation in both bipolar and unipolar depression, see Wolpert et al. (1990).*

see in later chapters, there are medications that can be effective in reducing or even eliminating these mood swings. We shall now, however, turn to the questions of how prevalent depression is in our society and who appears most vulnerable.

BIBLIOGRAPHY

American Psychiatric Association (1980). *Diagnostic and statistical manual of mental disorders* (3rd ed.). Washington, D.C.: Author.

Beck, A. T. (1967). *Depression: Clinical, experimental and theoretical aspects.* New York: Hoeber.

_____; Ward, C. H.; Mendelson, M.; Mock, J.; & Erbaugh, J. (1961). An inventory for measuring depression. *Archives of General Psychiatry*, 4, 561–71.

Cornell, D. G.; Suarez, R.; & Berent, S. (1984). Psychomotor retardation in melancholic and nonmelancholic depression: Cognitive and motor components. *Journal of Abnormal Psychology*, 93, 150–57.

Dauber, R. B. (1984). Subliminal psychodynamic activation in depression: On the role of autonomy issues in depressed college women. *Journal of Abnormal Psychology*, 93, 9–18.

DeAngelis, T. (1989). Mania, depression and genius. *American Psychological Association Monitor*, 20, no. 1, 1, 24.

Depue, R. A.; Slater, J. F.; Wolfsetter-Kausch, H.; Klein, D.; Goplerud, E.; & Farr, D. (1981). A behavioral paradigm for identifying persons at risk for bipolar depressive disorder: A conceptual framework and five validation studies. *Journal of Abnormal Psychology*, 90, 381–438.

Ellis, H. A. (1926). *A study of British genius.* Boston, Mass.: Houghton-Mifflin.

Fisch, H. U.; Frey, S.; & Hirsbrunner, H. P. (1983). Analyzing nonverbal behavior in depression. *Journal of Abnormal Psychology*, 92, 307–18.

Folkenberg, J. (1983, October). Using drugs to lift that dark veil of depression. *FDA Consumer*, 16–19.

Forgas, J. P.; Bower, G. H.; & Krantz, S. E. (1984). The influence of mood on perceptions of social interactions. *Journal of Experimental Social Psychology*, 20, 497–513.

Freud, S. (1959). *Mourning and melancholia.* In *Collected Papers*, vol. 4, 152–70. New York: Basic Books.

Gallagher, W. (1986, May). The dark affliction of mind and body. *Discover*, 7, no. 5, 66–76.

Goethe, Johann Wolfgang von (1774). *The Sorrows of Young Werther.* New York: Random House, 1971.

Hinz, L. D.; & Williamson, D. A. (1987). Bulimia and depression: A review of the affective variant hypothesis. *Psychological Bulletin*, 102, 150–58.

Jarrett, R. B.; & Weissenburger, J. E. (1990). Guilt in depressed outpatients. *Journal of Consulting and Clinical Psychology*, 58, 495–98.

Johnson, M. H.; & Magaro, P. A. (1987). Effects of mood and severity on memory processes in depression and mania. *Psychological Bulletin*, 101, 28–40.

Kocsis, J. H.; & Frances, A. J. (1987). A critical discussion of DSM-III dysthymic disorder. *American Journal of Psychiatry*, 144, 1534–42.

Kraepelin, E. (1913). *Textbook of psychiatry* (R. M. Barclay, trans.). Edinburgh: Livingstone.

Lewinsohn, P. M., & Teri, L. (1982). Selection of depressed and nondepressed subjects on the basis of self-report data. *Journal of Consulting and Clinical Psychology*, 50, 590–91.

McAllister, T. W. (1981). Cognitive functioning in the affective disorders. *Comprehensive Psychiatry*, 22, 572–86.

McMillan, M. J.; & Pihl, R. O. (1987). Premenstrual depression: A distinct entity. *Journal of Abnormal Psychology*, 96, 149–54.

Radloff, L. S. (1977). The CES-D Scale: A self-report depression scale for research in the general population. *Applied Psychological Measurement*, 1, 385–401.

Robbins, P. R., & Tanck, R. H. (1982). Further research using a psychological diary technique to investigate psychosomatic relationships. *Journal of Clinical Psychology*, 38, 356–59.

_____, & _____. (1987). A study of diurnal patterns of depressed mood. *Motivation and Emotion*, 11, 37–49.

Rosenthal, N. E.; Sack, D. A.; Gillin, J. C.; Lewy, A. J.; Goodwin, F. K.; Davenport, Y.; Mueller, P. S.; Newsome, D. A.; & Wehr, T. A. (1984). Seasonal affective disorder: A description of the syndrome and preliminary findings with light therapy. *Archives of General Psychiatry*, 41, 72–80.

Schmidt, J. M. (1981). The effects of subliminally presented anaclitic and introjective stimuli on normal young adults. Unpublished doctoral dissertation, University of Southern Mississippi.

Schwartz, G. E.; Fair, P. L.; Salt, P.; Mandel, M. R.; & Klerman, G. L. (1976). Facial muscle patterning to affective imagery in depressed and nondepressed subjects. *Science*, 192, 489–91.

Sedler, M. J. (1983). Falret's discovery: The origin of the concept of bipolar affective illness. *American Journal of Psychiatry*, 140, 1127–33.

Sirota, A. D., & Schwartz, G. E. (1982). Facial muscle patterning and lateralization during elation and depression imagery. *Journal of Abnormal Psychology*, 91, 25–34.

Sternberg, D. E., & Jarvik, M. E. (1976). Memory functions in depression: Improvement with antidepressant medication. *Archives of General Psychiatry*, 33, 219–24.

Velten, E. (1986). A laboratory task for induction of mood states. *Behaviour Research and Therapy*, 6, 473–82.

Wehr, T. A.; Sack, D. A.; & Rosenthal, N. E. (1987). Seasonal affective disorder with summer depression and winter hypomania. *American Journal of Psychiatry*, 144, 1602–3.

Wolpert, E. A.; Goldberg, J. F.; & Harrow, M. (1990). Rapid cycling in unipolar and bipolar affective disorders. *American Journal of Psychiatry*, 147, 725–28.

Zisook, S. (1988). Single case study: Cyclic 48-hour unipolar depression. *Journal of Nervous and Mental Disease*, 176, 53–56.

2. Depression in the United States

In pursuing our inquiry into depression, we are going to put on the hat of an epidemiologist—the statistically trained scientist who collects and analyzes data on diseases. In this role, we will ask such questions as: How many people in this country suffer from depression and which groups in the population seem to be at higher risk of becoming depressed? Are men or women more likely to become depressed? Does being in a minority group increase one's vulnerability? Does it make a difference whether one lives in an urban area or in the countryside? And what relation does the onset of depression bear to one's age? The answers to such questions will help us better understand the scope of the problem of depression in this country and identify groups of people at greater risk.

How does one estimate the number of people who suffer from depression? The problem is more difficult than it may seem. One possible approach would be to take a census of the nation's mental health centers and private practitioners, asking how many people are being treated for depression and who these people are. The problem with this approach is that a very large number of people who are depressed do not seek professional treatment. Moreover, the people who do seek treatment are not likely to be representative of the entire population of depressed people; they are likely to be more affluent and better educated. Minority groups will be underrepresented.

Probably the only way to estimate how many people are depressed in the United States is to go knocking on doors in our cities, towns and farms, to survey representative samples of our population and to ask questions that will accurately tell whether a person is depressed. And you have to do this in a way so that people will not slam the door in your face. After all, information about emotional health is sensitive.

The National Institute of Mental Health (NIMH) has made a concerted effort to address the problem. Researchers working under the auspices of NIMH have developed an interview guide – a series of questions that enables one to identify with reasonable accuracy people with different mental and emotional disorders. The technique has been validated by comparing the results obtained using the interview guide with the results from clinical evaluations. The interview guide was found to be acceptable for community surveys. Having said this, the technique should be viewed as a screening instrument and not as an ideal measure of depression. Like any other self-report measure of depression, it will classify some people who are actually clinically depressed as not depressed and some people who are not depressed as depressed. There is an error rate.

In large scale studies, researchers used the interview guide in selected communities in Connecticut, North Carolina, California, Maryland and Missouri. Thousands of people were interviewed in their homes. Preliminary results from these surveys indicated that about 5 percent of the adult population have suffered at one time or another from a major depression and 3 percent have experienced a protracted period of moderate depression (dysthymic disorder).[1] Translating these percentages into raw numbers, something like 9 million adult Americans have experienced a major depression and 5 million dysthymic disorder. At any given point in time, the number of persons experiencing depression would be less, though still numbering well into the millions.

A large majority of the cases of depression uncovered in these surveys were cases of unipolar depression. While the rates for experiencing a major depression were about five in one hundred, only one out of one hundred people interviewed reported ever experiencing a manic episode.

Studies carried out using the NIMH interviewing technique indicate that the chances of a person becoming depressed today are higher than they were in past generations. This conclusion is based on the findings that people who are now in their twenties are much more likely to report having experienced a depressive illness in their relatively short lives than people who are now senior citizens. If this is indeed the case, it is a striking observation.

There are, of course, problems in making comparisons between people

[1]*See Robins et al. (1984).*

at very different age ranges with different memories. One may raise questions about how reliable the memories of older people are about emotional troubles of much earlier years. Still, the apparently large increase in the rate of depression cannot be easily dismissed.

Why should people today be more prone to being depressed than people of past generations? While this is a tantalizing question, there are so many differences between the life-styles of today and earlier generations, that it is difficult to ascribe the apparent increase in depression to any one reason. One would be comparing an era of small towns to sprawling cities, traveling by train to traveling by jet, calculating numbers by hand to using computers. If I were forced to pick one reason to explain the apparent increase in depression, my candidate would be the breakdown of social support systems and most importantly, the family. The family has traditionally provided the individual with meaning and security. However, there has been a large increase in the number of families experiencing divorce and separation. Moreover, one is less likely to have one's extended family – aunts, uncles, cousins and grandparents – within hailing distance as might have been the case in the past. Today's life-style tends to scatter families. An individual may feel isolated, even rootless. In times of trouble and emotional stress, there may be no one close to turn to.

The idea that family ties, or to use a broader sociological term, *social integration*, has a relation to depressive behavior, is not a new one. One of the founding fathers of sociology, Emile Durkheim, reported in nineteenth-century France that persons who were more integrated into the society (e.g., married persons, persons coming from larger families) had lower suicide rates than those who were less integrated. I shall return to this theme – that social support has protective value against depression – in later chapters.

Sex Differences in Depression

When we compare groups of men and women we often find that women are more likely to be depressed. It should be stated that this is not always the case. For example, I once studied a sample of over 200 college students using a well-respected inventory to assess depression and found no difference between the male and female students.

However, when we examine the case records in treatment centers such as mental hospitals and outpatient clinics, we typically find that more of the cases diagnosed as depressed are women. Moreover, in community surveys, we usually find that more women than men report being depressed. For example, in a community study in Oregon, women were twice as likely as men to report being currently depressed.[2] The community surveys using the NIMH inteview guide have consistently found higher rates of unipolar depression in women. Interestingly, this was not the case for manic episodes.

A number of explanations have been offered to account for the higher rates of depression found in women. One theory is that women may be more biologically vulnerable to depression. It has been suggested that this vulnerability may relate in part to the reproductive system in women. Many women experience depressed reactions during the premenstrual phase of the menstrual cycle. Moreover, many women experience depressed reactions following the birth of a child. This *post partum* depression appears to be related to hormonal changes.

A second theory is that the cultural definition of being female permits women to more easily admit having emotional problems. From early on, males in our society are raised to be self-reliant and not to appear weak. The need to project a strong image may deter some men from admitting that they have a depressive problem and from seeking the help they need. According to this theory, men may have a higher rate of depression than is believed, but it is simply not reported.

Many men feel that if they express the fact that they are depressed to others, they may not only feel a loss of self-esteem, they may experience rejection. Constance Hammen and Stefanie Peters ran an experiment that suggests such fears are not groundless. Try the experiment on yourself. Read the following description of a young woman:

> Susan is 18 years old and a freshman in college. She was a good student in high school, well-adjusted, and got along well with her schoolmates. However, a couple of problems have developed since she started college. She is finding the course work quite a bit more difficult than she had expected, and lately it seems like her boyfriend from high school is losing interest in her.
>
> For the past few weeks, Susan has been feeling pretty down. She's feeling really miserable about what's been happening in her life and can't imagine that things will ever get any better. When she goes out with her friends or her

[2]*The Oregon studies cited in this book were carried out by Peter Lewinsohn and his coworkers. See Amenson & Lewinsohn (1981) for the discussion of gender differences in depression.*

boyfriend, she can't seem to shake her gloomy feelings and enjoy herself. Susan's been trying to keep up with her schoolwork, but she's falling farther and farther behind because most of the time she gets so discouraged and pessimistic that she gives up. The other day one of Susan's friends asked her if she wanted to have lunch together, but Susan said no because she hasn't really felt like eating lately and found that she had no appetite at all. Often she feels like there's no point in even getting up in the morning, and, in fact, Susan has been staying in bed longer and longer every morning. It seems like she just doesn't have any energy left for anything.[3]

Now ask yourself the following questions: How much would you like to have this person as an acquaintance? How much would you like her as a co-worker on a task? How much would you like her as a close friend?

Now go back and read the description of the person again, only this time, substitute a name like Bill or Jack for Susan, and girlfriend for boyfriend. When you finish, ask yourself the same three questions.

The subjects in the study carried out by Hammen and Peters were more likely to reject the person described when identified as a male than when identified as a female.

A third theory is that the role of women in our society often places them at a disadvantage, both economically and psychologically, leaving them in situations that increase their vulnerability to depressive reactions. Let's illustrate this idea with two case examples.

Tracy tells a story of being in an unhappy marriage. She was married shortly after high school graduation and had three children over the next six years. In the last two years her relationship with her husband has deteriorated, and he has been physically abusive. Tracy would like to leave him, but feels she can't. She has small children to support and sees no way of doing it. She feels dependent and powerless.

Denise is a single mother. She has near total responsibility for bringing in money from a job, keeping up the house and raising two children. This triple responsibility puts her in a perpetual time squeeze that creates high levels of stress, particularly when something goes wrong, like sickness in the children or herself. While both Tracy and Denise are vulnerable to depression because of their circumstances, research suggests that it is Tracy who may be the most vulnerable of the two. There are some studies—though research is not consistent on this point—that suggest that women who work and have multiple roles tend to be happier

[3]*Hammen & Peters (1977), pp. 995–96.*

than women who stay at home.[4] Multiple roles can certainly add interest to life and may decrease the chances of serious emotional letdown if something goes wrong in one area of life. Paid employment also decreases dependency, which is often a problem in depressive-prone people. The quality of the job and the degree to which it creates strains in other areas of a woman's life are, of course, important considerations in whether the job proves to be a plus or a minus for a woman's emotional health.

Rural-Urban Comparisons

One can make a case that the atmosphere of many cities is more turbulent than that of small towns and rural areas. Many big cities have serious problems with crime and drugs. They are congested, noisy and seem impersonal. In these respects, the stress-arousing potential of the city seems higher than that of rural areas. At the same time, the stress-buffering potential of family and close friends often found in integrated small communities may be diminished in the city. One might expect that these conditions could lead to higher rates of depression in urban areas.

Incidentally, ratings have been made for "stress levels" in American cities using such benchmarks as alcoholism, crime, suicide and divorce. Among cities rated high in stress are Reno, Las Vegas, Miami, and Los Angeles.[5] But one also finds high on the list Little Rock, Arkansas, and Odessa, Texas. Looking for less stress? According to the ratings, you might try Grand Forks, North Dakota, or Rochester, Minnesota. Is there something about warm climates that creates turmoil or are people up north too chilled by the snow and ice to get excited?

The idea that one might find less depression in low-stress environments receives some support from research conducted in close-knit, less technologically advanced communities. For example, researchers studying a primitive tribe in New Guinea in 1984 found little evidence of depression or suicide. A study of the Amish people in Lancaster County, Pennsylvania, also found low rates of unipolar depression.[6] Using the

---

[4]*See, for example, Cochrane & Stopes-Roe (1981).*

[5]*See Levine (1988). The stress ratings are based on social indicators, not the perceptions of the residents, which might yield a different picture.*

[6]*See Seligman (1988), p. 50. The observations in New Guinea were carried out on the Kaluli tribe by Edward Schieffelin. The studies on the Amish were conducted by Janice Egeland and her colleagues. See Egeland & Hostetter (1983).*

household survey technique, researchers have compared rates of depression in several urban and rural American communities. Their findings indicate that depression is indeed more frequent in urban environments.

Here is an illustrative study. A research team surveyed five counties in North Carolina.[7] One of the counties—Durham County—was part of a major urban center containing several well-known universities and an industrial park. The four rural counties contained no major industries and were described as representative of the rural South.

Carefully chosen samples of people in these communities were interviewed using the NIMH interview guide. The results? Reports of current major depressive episodes were *three times* as frequent in the urban county. When the researchers controlled statistically for a number of important social and demographic factors, such as sex, education, race and selective migration, they continued to find a substantial difference in the rates of depression between the urban and rural areas. Results such as this lead to the conclusion that urban life is associated with a higher risk of depression.

Depression in Members of Minority Groups

Let's turn our attention to the question of whether depression is more likely to occur among members of minority groups. Our focus will be on three of America's largest minority groups—African, Hispanic and Asian Americans.

In considering the potential risk for depression among these minority groups, we might start with the observation that African Americans and Hispanics are likely to be economically poorer than non–Hispanic whites. The same is likely to be true for recent immigrants from Southeast Asia. These groups, then, have a higher chance of living in poorer, more crime-ridden neighborhoods. They may also be subjected to prejudice based on racial and ethnic bias. In addition, African Americans have a higher rate of single parent families than other groups, which brings additional burdens. All of these factors might lead one to speculate that at least some minority groups are exposed to relatively high levels of en-

[7]*Blazer et al. (1985). The statistically controlled analyses suggested that the depression rate in the urban areas was twice as high as in the rural areas.*

vironmental stressors, which might be reflected in higher rates of depression.

Is this deduction correct? Let's look at the research, beginning with studies of depression among African Americans. If we consider only *depressed mood*, that transitory feeling that comes and goes, there is evidence that African Americans tend to experience this more than whites. Researchers presenting words describing moods, such as *lost, tormented, forlorn* and *rejected*, to representative samples of the population have found that African Americans were more likely than whites to report that these words described their feelings.[8] However, the same findings also held true when the researchers compared poorer people to richer people, and unskilled laborers to professionals. People who do not "have it made" feel less hopeful.

If we go beyond mood and consider depression as a group of symptoms, the differences between African Americans and white Americans disappear. One line of evidence comes from research that used a well-known psychological test, the Minnesota Multiphasic Personality Inventory (MMPI). This test contains two scales of particular interest for our inquiry: a measure of depression and a measure of the tendency towards hypomania. Many samples of African Americans and whites have been studied using the MMPI, and the results show little difference on the depression scale. There is some tendency for African Americans to score higher on the hypomania scale, however, which might indicate higher vulnerability to bipolar depression.

Another line of evidence comes from community studies in which comparisons were made between African American and white persons in terms of reported depression. In general, these studies have found rather similar rates of depression for African Americans and whites, which is consistent with the MMPI findings.

The suggestion raised by the MMPI studies that African Americans might be more vulnerable to bipolar depression has not been fully resolved. In two large community studies, no appreciable differences in the rate of bipolar depression were found for African Americans and whites, but in one community study carried out in St. Louis, African Americans did report a higher rate of bipolar disorder.[9]

There are reasons to suspect that Hispanic Americans, particularly

---

[8]*Lubin et al. (1988).*
[9]*See Robins et al. (1984). The data for manic episodes are presented in table 7, p. 956.*

recent immigrants, might be vulnerable to depression. Writing about Puerto Ricans, for example, Lillian Comas-Díaz stated in a 1981 article that they have "the highest degree of poverty and unemployment among minorities in the United States mainland. . . . This condition may be a major factor in relation to the feelings of marginality and helplessness that are expressed by a large proportion of Puerto Ricans living in the continental United States. As part of the myriad of stressful situations encountered in a new reality, Puerto Ricans who migrate to the mainland face culture shock, poverty, and powerlessless."[10] Comas-Díaz theorized that the Puerto Rican woman is especially vulnerable because she "has been socialized into a powerless position. . . . Her cultural background emphasizes passivity, helplessness, non-assertiveness and dependency."[11]

This analysis presents a rather bleak picture, pointing toward a high rate of depression in Puerto Ricans, especially women. There is at least one study that appears to support this contention.[12] However, I am not sure one can generalize these observations to all Hispanic Americans. Indeed, the most comprehensive study I am aware of that was carried out on a large sample of Mexican Americans living in two Los Angeles communities points to a quite different conclusion. The rates for most mental disorders studied were generally similar for Mexican Americans and non–Hispanic whites. The lifetime prevalence of major depressive episodes was *lower* for Mexican Americans than for non–Hispanic whites.

There were some very interesting findings reported for Hispanic women. In the younger age range Hispanic women were *much less* likely to be depressed than young non–Hispanic white women. However, when the researchers looked at Hispanic women over 40, they found a relatively large number of women who reported long-lasting, moderate levels of depression (dysthymic disorder).[13]

One wonders what is it about growing up in a Mexican American family that offers young women protection against depressive reactions? Is it the protection of a close-knit, extended family, where one has many links to other people? Is it the immersion in religion that often assumes a predominant place in Hispanic culture? Is there more certainty in the

[10]*Comas-Díaz (1981), p. 627.*
[11]*Comas-Díaz (1981), p. 627.*
[12]*See Torres-Matrullo (1976).*
[13]*See Karno et al. (1987). For a discussion of ethnic comparisons, see p. 700.*

future roles of young women, with less pressure toward career achievement?

One also wonders what happens in later life that breaks down this early protection leaving Mexican American women more vulnerable toward a protracted malaise. Is it, as Comas-Díaz suggests, being locked into a position of dependency with feelings of powerlessness? We need more research to be sure.

When we turn to Asian Americans, it is difficult to give a clear answer to the question of the prevalence of depression. There are over 3,500,000 Asian Americans in the United States, including about 700,000 refugees admitted to the country since the mid-1970s. The language barrier makes it particularly difficult to obtain accurate figures for the prevalence of depression in the refugee population. The use of interpreters can lead to misleading conclusions because of the subtlety of language used in the description of psychological states. An example of the errors that can result from the use of a translator is provided in an article by Luis Marcos.

A clinician wanted information from a Chinese-speaking patient. He asked, "What kinds of moods have you been in recently?" The interpreter turned to the patient and asked, "How have you been feeling?" The patient replied to the interpreter, "No, I don't have any more pain, my stomach is now fine, and I can eat much better since I take the medication." The interpreter said to the clinician, "He says that he feels fine, no problems."[14]

Notwithstanding the difficulties involved, researchers who have studied the mental health of the refugees from Southeast Asia report that they have observed a rather high level of psychiatric problems among the immigrants. The dislocations resulting from the exodus from countries in Southeast Asia appears to have taken a heavy emotional toll.

In contrast to the refugees, the more established Asian American populations, the Chinese and Japanese, have a reputation for being well adjusted. There is little question but that Chinese and Japanese Americans are less likely than whites to use both inpatient and outpatient mental health facilities. For example, the admission rates to California state mental hospitals are far lower for Japanese and Chinese Americans than for whites. The same holds true in Hawaii.

These statistics, however, may be misleading as indicators of the true

[14]*Marcos (1979), p. 173.*

extent of psychological distress, including depression, among Asian Americans. It seems likely that many Asian Americans find other ways of dealing with their emotional problems than seeking the assistance of mental health professionals. In writing about mental illness in Asian Americans, David and Stanley Sue observed that the "amount of stigma or shame associated with emotional difficulties is probably much greater among Asian American groups. Mental illness in a family member is considered a failure of the family system itself. For Eastern more than for Western families, the failure or weakness of an individual is considered a disgrace to the family unit. . . . [Researchers] reported that the stigma of mental illness in Asian Americans remains so great that, even among individuals of the third and fourth generation, there is hesitation to admit to psychological problems."[15]

Researchers have reported that Asian Americans seem willing to describe their problems in terms of bodily complaints—headaches, fatigue, insomnia, dizziness and heart palpitations—but are reluctant to admit to demoralized psychological states. This denial of an emotional problem may even persist into treatment. Given this cultural tradition, which would lead to underreporting of the problem, it would be difficult to make an accurate estimate of the prevalence of depressive problems among Asian Americans.

With this caveat about the uncertainty of depression among Asian Americans, it seems fair to conclude that to date there is little evidence to suggest that depression is more frequent among members of minority groups than in the general population.

Age at Onset of Depression

At what age do people become depressed? Is it likely to begin in early childhood? Adolescence? Young adulthood? Is the age of onset of depression the same for men and women?

To answer these questions, researchers have been carrying out studies with relatively large numbers of people. For example, in Oregon over 2,000 people who had shown some evidence of depression on psychological screening tests were interviewed in detail about current and

[15]*Sue and Sue (1987), p. 480.*

past episodes of depression.[16] About 1,000 of the people were diagnosed as having at least one current or past episode of unipolar depression.

In the interviews, the researchers tried to ascertain the time at which the first episode of depression occurred. They found that the risk of developing depression in childhood was *very low*. Before we accept this conclusion as gospel, however, we must point out that there have been real difficulties in diagnosing depression in children.

As an anchoring point in what has been an area of controversy, we should note that children are being treated today in psychiatric hospitals for depression. Using the benchmarks described in the American Psychiatric Association's *Diagnostic and Statistical Manual*, children have been diagnosed as having major depressions and are being treated using psychotherapy and antidepressant drugs.

What is a young child who is diagnosed as having a major depression like? Here are some excerpts from a case study presented by Javad Kashani and his colleagues.

The depressed child, a five-year-old boy named Mike, became a matter of considerable concern to his teacher "when he told her that he wanted to 'kill himself and die.' The teacher found him to be sad, worried, overactive, restless and irritable. He had feelings of self-reproach, self-blame, and hopelessness about the future and had difficulty in concentrating and following rules." Mike had physical complaints such as stomachaches and pains in his legs and arms. He was also fatigued. His mother reported that he had crying spells, was irritable and had a poor appetite.

When Mike was interviewed by the researcher, he did not smile, but appeared solemn. He said he didn't like himself and that nobody liked him. When he was asked what was going to happen to him when he became a big man, he replied, "I'll be dead."[17]

Mike is a depressed child, not difficult to recognize as such. So, too, are other children in psychiatric hospitals being treated with drugs and psychotherapy. When we move away from such severe cases, however,

---

[16]See *Lewinsohn et al. (1986). Subsequent reports using the NIMH Interview Schedule have noted that the adolescent and young adult years are important periods for the development of both unipolar depression and bipolar illness with the latter tending to occur somewhat earlier. See Burke, et al. (1990).*

[17]*Kashani et al. (1986), p. 1141.*

the problem becomes murkier.[18] It is hard to say how many children in this country should be considered depressed.

One of the reasons for this uncertainty is that the clinicians and researchers who have studied depression in children have disagreed about the very nature of childhood depression. In describing the disorder, some writers have included symptoms that go well beyond those listed in the *Diagnostic and Statistical Manual* for adults. They have interpreted a number of troublesome behaviors in children as "masking depression," behaviors that disguise an underlying depression. Behaviors as wide-ranging as hyperactivity, aggressiveness, delinquency, temper tantrums, boredom and restlessness have been cited as evidence of depression. In a paper on childhood depression, Monroe Lefkowitz and Edward Tesiny observed that such a "catalogue of symptoms must, at one time or another, encompass all children."[19]

At the other extreme, it has been argued that much of what has been called depression in childhood is really transitory problems in development—problems that often disappear as children grow up. An example would be poor appetite, a symptom of depression in adults. One study identified a number of children at age six with poor appetites. By age nine the problem in most of the children had disappeared.[20] It would be stretching things to infer that these children had been depressed.

If we try using psychological screening inventories in which children report depressive symptoms similar to the inventories used by adults, the situation is not helped appreciably. The meaning of these test scores is not all that clear. In one study, for example, researchers used a children's depression inventory to try to distinguish between children in a clinic diagnosed as depressed and children diagnosed as having "conduct" disorders such as truancy or overaggressiveness. The test misclassified about two-thirds of the children.[21]

---

[18]*The difficulty of identifying children with subclinical levels of depression was highlighted in a study carried out by Reed Larson and his co-workers. They monitored the moods and behavior of 483 fifth- and ninth-graders for a week, comparing the behavior of children who scored high on a children's depression inventory with those who did not. They reported, "In general, we were struck by how few associations there were between depression and how children and young adolescents experienced the different contexts of their lives. Outwardly, the daily patterns of depressed children and adolescents are quite like those of nondepressed peers." Larson et al. (1990).*

[19]*Lefkowitz & Tesiny (1980), p. 43.*

[20]*See Macfarlane et al. (1954).*

[21]*See Carey et al. (1987).*

In another example, researchers administered a children's depression inventory to children in the schools of four rural communities. To estimate the prevalence of depression, the researchers used "cutoff" scores suggested by the developers of the instrument. A score above a certain number was supposed to indicate the likelihood of depression. Using these recommended cutoff scores for identifying depression, the researchers would have come up with the astonishing figure that 46 percent of the children in the community were depressed.[22] This figure, of course, is ludicrous and just emphasizes the fact that we simply do not yet have accurate ways of identifying depression in young children that can be applied to large samples with confidence.

In reviewing the state of the art, Mary Kerr and her colleagues likened recent attempts to conceptualize and measure depression in children to the story of the blind man examining the elephant. Because of these troublesome problems in definition and measurement, I think it is fair to say that we not as yet have a satisfactory estimate of the number of children who are depressed in this country. One of the reasons for this uncertainty is that depression in children is not always easy to recognize. It is not difficult to spot a "problem child" who bullies his playmates, has recurrent nightmares or sets fires at home, but a child who seems lonely or sad may not be viewed as being all that unusual. The child may be described as "quiet" or "shy," rather than depressed. The parents or teacher may not identify a depressive problem if it exists, and young children should not be expected to diagnose themselves.

While we may not often recognize depression in young children—either because it occurs infrequently, as suggested by the Oregon study, or because we are not sophisticated enough to identify it when it does occur—the situation is quite different for adolescents. The problem of suicide among teenagers, for example, has received a great deal of publicity and for good reason. Suicide is the second leading cause of death among people in the 15 to 24 age range.

A survey carried out in 1988 on over 11,000 teenagers revealed some rather startling statistics.[23] Four out of 10 girls and 1 out of 5 boys said they have seriously thought about committing suicide at some time during their lives. Most of the young people indicated that they would find it difficult to tell their parents or teachers about these thoughts.

[22]*See Doerfler et al. (1988).*
[23]*See Landers (1988).*

One comes across grim stories of teenage suicide in the newspapers. I read a very sad account of two teenage girls who entered into a suicide pact. The girls told their friends that they wanted to find a gun. When they found one, they went to an area in the local park and killed themselves. One of the girls was known to have suffered from emotional problems.

How extensive is depression among adolescents? William Reynolds surveyed high schools using a battery of self-report measures of depression and reported that he found levels of moderate to severe depression running in about 11 to 17 percent of the students. Correcting for the possibility that self-report inventories may overestimate the extent of depression when compared to interviews conducted by trained clinicians, it still looks as if depression in adolescents is a widespread problem.

Psychologists studying "loneliness" have found that these very unpleasant feelings, which often coincide with depression, peak during the teenage years. Adolescents are noted for their gregariousness but frequently feel lonely and sometimes alienated.

Turning to college students, Roland Tanck and I included in our diary the questions, "Did you feel depressed today?, and if *yes*, what do you think was causing these depressed feelings?" In perusing the students' responses, we noticed that while on occasion the students were at a loss to identify the cause of their depressed moods, they usually offered a reason, and often a specific event. Frequently, the students attributed their depressed feelings to problems relating to school work. A few examples of such responses were, "I feel very behind in my school work as though I will never catch up," "Without a doubt—the chemistry exam," and "Big test that I did poorly on."

The students pointed to relationships as another source of depressed feelings. Sometimes, the depressed feelings were caused by problems in a romantic relationship. For example, "He is interested in someone else more than me," or "A problem with a boyfriend." Sometimes there was friction in a relationship. Some examples are, "A fight with a friend," or "An unpleasant conversation with the girl upstairs." And sometimes there was the possibility of a breakup of relationships: "I thought too much about two good friends who are transferring next semester."

At times, the students identified the source of their depressed feelings not as events, but as their own thought processes. Sometimes the students spent time looking within themselves, questioning their own performance. "My lack of motivation to do things," or "I'm wasting too much time." Sometimes they thought about the future and felt uncertain about where they were going: "I was wondering where my life is leading." And occasionally, there was a vague feeling of concern, such as "I was worrying about life in general."

Reading through our collection of student diaries leaves one with the impression that a great many college students experience periods of mild to moderate depression. Using a depression inventory, we estimated that about 14 percent of the students in our research project were moderately depressed.

The statistics from the Oregon study point to the conclusion that the risk of becoming depressed increases sharply in the late adolescent and young adult years. For males, the risk seems to peak by the early twenties and holds pretty much constant until it begins to decline in the later years of life. The years of higher education, of starting a career, of developing relationships, of marriage and starting a family—these years of ever-increasing responsibility are the years when depression is most likely to occur in men.

Kevin, a young musician whose career ambitions had been side-tracked by the pressures of an early marriage, is an example of this age-related risk in men. From an early age, Kevin had hoped to become a pianist. In his second year of college, he met Julie, an art student, fell in love, married and within a year became a father. His musical studies slipped into the background as he took jobs that were unrelated to music in order to support his family. He waited on tables, tried selling real estate, then took a job as a bank teller. The birth of his second child made it still harder to seriously resume his studies. The press of responsibilities and the fading of his dreams posed an emotional strain to both Kevin and his wife. Kevin became irritable and difficult to talk to. He became morose and withdrawn. Eventually, he entered therapy for depression.

Interestingly, the Oregon researchers report a somewhat different pattern for women. The risk of becoming depressed does not reach its highest point in the young adult years for women, but continues to rise, reaching a peak near the age of fifty. This difference in peak age of onset of depression may reflect traditional differences in sex roles. For example, society has placed a higher premium on physical attractiveness in women than in men and the fading of physical beauty may have more of an emotional impact on women. In addition, the responsibilities and satisfactions that come with childrearing traditionally provide a great deal of meaning in the lives of women, and when these diminish as children leave home, many women experience an emotional letdown and a sense of emptiness in their lives.

Women differ greatly in the way they adapt to these role transitions. Many women find that diminished family responsibilities and increased time for themselves provide an opportunity to fulfill longstanding ambitions. Janice, for example, always wanted to write children's books and now has the time to do so. Ellen always wanted to travel and decided to take a tour of Europe with her husband. In contrast, Rose, who was a housewife for many years, found herself with few meaningful things to do after the children were gone. She did not want to incur the risks involved with reentering the job market and was at loose ends. She was caught in what has been called the "empty nest syndrome" and would appear to be the most vulnerable of the three women.

As is true for men, there is a decline in the onset of depression in women during the later years of life. In reflecting on these trends, it appears that the most likely time for the onset of a depressive illness is the prime time of life. What may be one's best years in terms of drive, energy and capability may also be one's most vulnerable years for becoming depressed.

Depression Among the Elderly

Some years ago I was a member of an organization of volunteers — physicians, nurses, psychologists and social workers, which provided free health services to people who did not have easy access to medical services. My assignment along with another psychologist was to offer therapy to the residents of a large public housing project for the elderly. Many of the residents came to our weekly evening clinic, but only a few people ever asked for an appointment with a therapist.

At the time I was surprised by the apparently low prevalence of emotional problems among the residents. In reading articles on aging, I was struck by all of the things that can go wrong: chronic illness, slowdown in mental acuity, financial deprivation, widowhood, loss of friends, and so on. Given these conditions, I expected to encounter a lot of emotional problems, particularly depression. However, in the senior citizens' apartment complex, that did not seem to be the case.

The senior citizens' housing complex offered a wide range of social and recreational activities. The complex was not just a roof over one's head; it was a place to live and socialize. Perhaps it was these opportunities for an active life-style that helped keep psychological distress to a minimum.

Consider a contrasting situation. I once acted as a consultant to another senior citizens' facility, a very large metropolitan nursing home. The residents were not as well off physically as the residents in the housing complex, nor did they enjoy the same quality of life in terms of housing, social life and recreational activities. With the aid of the institution's nursing staff, we carried out a study of psychological problems among the residents of the nursing home and found evidence that about 15 percent of the residents experienced at least one depressive episode during a six-week observational period.

These two isolated observations point to a conclusion that is buttressed by considerable research. The physical health and social environment of senior citizens can make a difference in whether they are likely to experience depression. Good health, a stimulating environment, and social relationships are important in maintaining a positive attitude and outlook.

When we pose the question "What is the prevalence of depression in the elderly?" we encounter some difficulties. A significant number of elderly people suffer from brain disorders such as Alzheimer's disease and unless some care in diagnosis is made, it is possible to confuse some symptoms of depression with brain dysfunction. Another problem is that elderly people all too often learn of the death of family members and close friends and experience the grief that comes with such loss. Grief and depression are not the same, but may appear similar and can easily be confused. It is quite possible that when the researcher looks for the symptoms of depression, he or she may find them, even though the person is not clinically depressed.

Elderly people typically see their physician for problems rather than consulting a mental health specialist. When they see a physician, research suggests that the physician might not diagnose a depression and the problem could go untreated. In a study of a sample of elderly patients at a Veterans Administration Hospital, only 2 of 23 depressed elderly patients were correctly identified by the house staff as depressed.[24]

[24]*Rapp et al. (1988).*

All of these considerations then lead to some caution in making hard and fast estimates of the prevalence of depression in the elderly. With these problems in mind, some community surveys suggest that about 10 to 18 percent of older adults experience symptoms of depression.[25] However, most of these people probably are not experiencing a major depression. Some estimates of the prevalence of a major depression among the elderly run on the order of 3 to 6 percent. The Oregon study further suggests that such depression is relatively infrequent in older people.

Depression is more likely to be a problem in unmarried elderly people, which may reflect the fact that loneliness is linked to depression. The person without strong social ties is vulnerable.

An example is Kathy Biggs, an elderly, retired librarian. Kathy led a quiet, fairly solitary life in a suburban community. She read a great deal, worked in her garden and spent a lot of time with a lifelong friend, Joan. Joan died suddenly and unexpectedly. It was a terrible blow to Kathy. The loss, coupled with increasing physical disabilities of her own, left Kathy alone and isolated. Her quiet world had been turned upside down and she had no one to turn to. She began to experience many of the symptoms of depression.

Some studies, though not all, indicate that the risk of depression is higher among seniors in the less affluent stratas of society. Being caught in a daily economic squeeze and not being able to do much about it can create constant psychological pressures, which may lead to depressed reactions.

In this chapter I have presented some statistics about the prevalence of depression in the United States. The figures presented depend on the methods used to obtain the information, and these methods are far from perfect.

Still, it is very clear that the problem of depression is widespread. We are talking about millions of adults who have experienced moderate to severe levels of depression and a problem that happens to all of the groups that make up our society. And we are talking about a problem that is likely to arise in the prime of life.

---

[25]*For example, Murrell et al. (1983). In this community study, which used the Center for Epidemiologic Studies Depression Scale to measure depression, 14 percent of the men studied and 18 percent of the women studied were considered depressed.*

BIBLIOGRAPHY

Amenson, C. S., & Lewinsohn, P. M. (1981). An investigation into the observed sex difference in prevalence of unipolar depression. *Journal of Abnormal Psychology*, 90, 1–13.

Barnett, P. A., & Gotlib, I. H. (1988). Psychosocial functioning and depression: Distinguishing among antecendents, concomitants, and consequences. *Psychological Bulletin*, 104, 97–126.

Blazer, D.; George, L. K.; Landerman, R.; Pennybacker, M.; Melville, M. L.; Woodbury, M.; Manton, K. G.; Jordan, K.; & Locke, B. (1985). Psychiatric disorders: A rural/urban comparison. *Archives of General Psychiatry*, 42, 651–56.

Burke, K. C.; Burke, J. D., Jr.; Regier, D. A.; & Rae, D. S. (1990). Age at onset of selected mental disorders in five community populations. *Archives of General Psychiatry*, 47, 511–18.

Burnam, M. A.; Hough, R. L.; Escobar, J. I,; Karno, M.; Timbers, D. M.; Telles, C. A.; & Locke, B. Z. (1987). Six-month prevalence of specific psychiatric disorder among Mexican Americans and non–Hispanic Whites in Los Angeles. *Archives of General Psychiatry*, 44, 687–94.

Carey, M. P.; Faulstich, M. E.; Gresham, F. M.; Ruggiero, L.; & Enyart, P. (1987). Children's Depression Inventory: Construct validity across clinical and nonreferred (control) populations. *Journal of Consulting and Clinical Psychology*, 55, 755–61.

Cochrane, R., & Stopes-Roe, M. (1981). Women, marriage, employment and mental health, *British Journal of Psychiatry*, 139, 373–81.

Comas-Díaz, L. (1981). Effects of cognitive and behavioral group treatment on the depressive symptomatology of Puerto Rican women. *Journal of Consulting and Clinical Psychology*, 49, 627–32.

Doerfler, L. A.; Felner, R. D.; Rowlison, R. T.; Raley, P. A.; & Evans, E. (1988). Depression in children and adolescents: A comparative analysis of the utility and construct validity of two assessment measures. *Journal of Consulting and Clinical Psychology*, 56, 769–72.

Durkheim, E. (1966). *Suicide.* New York: Free Press.

Egeland, J. A., & Hostetter, A. M. (1983). Amish study: I. Affective disorders among the Amish, 1976–1980. *American Journal of Psychiatry*, 140, 56–61.

Hammen, C. L., & Peters, S. D. (1977). Differential responses to male and female depressive reactions. *Journal of Consulting and Clinical Psychology*, 45, 994–1001.

Hopkins, J.; Marcus, M.; & Campbell, S. B. (1984). Postpartum depression: A critical review. *Psychological Bulletin*, 95, 498–515.

Karno, M.; Hough, R. L.; Burnam, A.; Escobar, J. I.; Timbers, D. M.; Santana, F.; & Boyd, J. H. (1987). Lifetime prevalence of specific psychiatric disorders among Mexican Americans and non–Hispanic Whites in Los Angeles. *Archives of General Psychiatry*, 44, 695–701.

Kashani, J. H.; Holcomb, W. R.; & Orvaschel, H. (1986). Depression and depressive symptoms in preschool children from the general population. *American Journal of Psychiatry*, 143, 1138–43.

Kendell, R. E.; Wainwright, S.; Hailey, A.; & Shannon, B. (1976). The influence of childbirth on psychiatric morbidity. *Psychological medicine*, 6, 297–302.

Kerr, M. M.; Hoier, T. S.; & Versi, M. (1987). Methodological issues in childhood depression: A review of the literature. *American Journal of Orthopsychiatry*, 57, 193–98.

Landers, S. (1988, November 30). Survey verifies teen risk-taking. *American Psychological Association Monitor*, 30.

Larson, R. W.; Rafaelli, M.; Richards, M. H.; Ham, M.; & Jewell, L. (1990). Ecology of depression in late childhood and early adolescence: A profile of daily states and activities. *Journal of Abnormal Psychology*, 99, 92–102.

Lewinsohn, P. M.; Duncan, E. M.; Stanton, A. K.; & Hautzinger, M. (1986). Age at first onset for nonbipolar depression. *Journal of Abnormal Psychology*, 95, 378–83.

Lubin, B.; Zuckerman, M.; Breytspraak, L. M.; Bull, N. C.; Gumbhir, A. K.; & Rinck, C. M. (1988). Affects, demographic variables, and health. *Journal of Clinical Psychology*, 44, 131–41.

Macfarlane, J. W.; Allen, L.; & Honzik, M. P. (1954). *Developmental study of the behavior problems of normal children between twenty-one months and fourteen years.* Berkeley: University of California Press.

Marcos, L. R. (1979). Effects of interpreters on the evaluation of psychopathology in non–English speaking patients. *American Journal of Psychiatry*, 136, 171–74.

Murrell, S. A.; Himmelfarb, S.; & Wright, K. (1983). Prevalence of depression and its correlates in older adults. *American Journal of Epidemiology*, 117, 173–85.

Nolen-Hoeksema, S. (1987). Sex differences in unipolar depression: Evidence and theory. *Psychological Bulletin*, 101, 259–82.

Phifer, J. F., & Murrell, S. A. (1986). Etiologic factors in the onset of depressive symptoms in older adults. *Journal of Abnormal Psychology*, 95, 282–91.

Quesada, G. M.; Spears, W.; & Ramos, P. (1978). Interracial depressive epidemiology in the Southwest. *Journal of Health and Social Behavior*, 19, 77–85.

Rapp, S. R.; Parisi, S. A.; Walsh, D. A.; & Wallace, C. E. (1988). Detecting depression in elderly medical inpatients. *Journal of Consulting and Clinical Psychology*, 56, 509–13.

Reynolds, W. M., & Coats, K. I. (1982). Depression in adolescents: Incidence, depth, and correlates. Paper presented at 10th International Congress, International Association of Child and Adolescent Psychiatry and Allied Professions, Dublin, Ireland.

Robbins, P. R.; Kleh, J.; & Meyersburg, H. A. (1973). Psychological problems in the care of the institutionalized aged: A look at D. C. Village. *Medical Annals of the District of Columbia, 42,* 385–89.

Robins, L. N.; Helzer, J. E.; Croughan, J.; & Ratcliff, K. S. (1981). National Institute of Mental Health Diagnostic Interview Schedule: Its history, characteristics and validity. *Archives of General Psychiatry, 38,* 381–89.

_____; _____; Wiessman, M. M.; Orvaschel, H.; Gruenberg, E.; Burke, J. D.; & Regier, D. A. (1984). Lifetime prevalence of specific psychiatric disorders in three sites. *Archives of General Psychiatry, 41,* 949–58.

Seligman, M. E. P. (1988, October). Boomer blues. *Psychology Today, 22,* 50–55.

Sue, D., & Sue, S. (1987). Cultural factors in the clinical assessment of Asian Americans. *Journal of Consulting and Clinical Psychology, 55,* 479–87.

Torres-Matrullo, C. (1976). Acculturation and psychopathology among Puerto Rican women in mainland United States. *American Journal of Orthopsychiatry, 46,* 710–19.

Westermeyer, J.; Vang, T. F.; & Neider, J. (1983). A comparison of refugees using and not using a psychiatric service: An analysis of DSM III criteria and self-rating scales in cross-cultural context. *Journal of Operational Psychiatry, 14,* 36–41.

3. The Biological Bases of Depression

I remember looking through a textbook on abnormal psychology written for undergraduate students in the 1950s and being struck by the effort to explain the causes of mental illness in purely psychological terms. Manic depressive disorder and schizophrenia were viewed as exaggerations of normal psychological tendencies. Little attention was given to biological bases for these emotional and mental disturbances. One of the reasons for this approach was that scientists looking for biological links to these disorders had as yet not been able to find very much.

In more recent years, the situation has changed dramatically. The development of antidepressant drugs and the discovery that many clinically depressed people have imbalances in the neurotransmitters in the brain have spurred intensive interest in the biological bases of depression. The pendulum has swung to the point that one hears people talk about depression as a biological illness.

With the perspective that increasingly sophisticated research provides, it now seems likely that both biological and psychological factors play major roles in depressive disorders. The task that lies ahead for scientists will be to integrate the findings from both disciplines to provide a comprehensive model that will best explain depression.

What I will attempt to do in this chapter is to present thumbnail sketches of some of the important findings showing biological bases for depression. We will look first at the influence of heredity on depression. Then we will consider the role of the neurotransmitters in depression, the possibilities for a laboratory test for depression, and the links between depression and physiological measures of sleep. I will conclude with a discussion of depression and the immune system.

Many diseases "run in families." Some examples that come to mind are allergies, hypertension, Alzheimer's disease and schizophrenia. When we say that an illness "runs in families" we simply mean that some-one in a family in which one person has been afflicted is more likely to develop the problem than someone in a family where there is no history of the disease. It does not mean that everyone in the family will develop the problem or that the onset of the disorder is inevitable. We are saying that the risk is higher.

When we observe such family patterns, we often suspect that there is some genetic basis for what we see. This may not always be the case, for environmental conditions can trigger both physical and emotional problems and members of a family are usually exposed to a similar en-vironment. A high level of stress, a pattern of poverty, or destructive parenting practices can affect all exposed persons. Still, the possibility of a hereditary basis for an illness is an obvious place to start looking when we observe familial patterns of illness.

Depression has some tendency to run in families. If someone in a family is clinically depressed, a very close relative—son or daughter, sister or brother or parent—has a higher risk than someone in the general population of developing the problem. Some statistics that have been reported suggest that the likelihood of a depressive episode is about 15 percent for persons who have close family members who are depressed.[1] In evaluating these figures, it is well to keep in mind the surveys that reported the prevalence of depression in the general population: esti-mates are that about 5 percent of the population has experienced a major depression, and 3 percent, dysthymic disorder. So the risk for a person in a family where there is a depressed case appears higher than for the general population.

When we move away from very close relatives to more distant rela-tives, the likelihood of a depressive illness occurring decreases. Among such relatives as aunts, uncles and grandparents, the risk of depression runs around 7 percent, which is close to the risk of anyone in the general population.[2]

The fact that depression does run in families suggests the possibility of a genetic basis for the disorder. Is this the case? One of the best ways to establish that heredity plays a role in a disorder is to carry out studies that use the twin study method. In such studies, one compares the con-

[1]*Sargent (1986), p. 7.*
[2]*Sargent (1986), p. 7.*

cordance of depression in identical twins (monozygotic twins) and fraternal twins (dizygotic twins). The reasoning behind such studies goes something like this: Monozygotic twins have exactly the same heredity, coming from the same fertilized ovum. Dizygotic twins happen to be born at the same time and share a common environment, but come from different fertilized ovums. Such twins have the same hereditary makeup as any other pair of siblings. If heredity plays a role in depression, we would expect to find more cases among monozygotic twins than dizygotic twins in which when one member of a set becomes depressed, the other member also becomes depressed. And this is just what we find in research.

An example of this type of study was carried out by a research team in Australia. The team, led by Kenneth Kendler, mailed questionnaires to people listed on the Australian Twin Register. They received about 4,000 replies from both members of twin sets. The questionnaire included items that asked about depressive symptoms. The researchers found much more similarity in the responses of the monozygotic twins to these items than in the responses of the dizygotic twins.

The twin study method has also been applied to the study of patients who are clinically depressed. Statistics reported for the concordance for unipolar depression indicate that if one member of a pair of monozygotic twins is diagnosed as having a unipolar depression, in 40 percent of the cases, the other twin will have the condition also. The concordance for dizygotic twins was 11 percent.[3]

While these twin studies clearly point to an important role for heredity in the cause of unipolar depression, they also indicate that environmental factors are significant. If heredity were totally determinative, both members of monozygotic twin sets would invariably come down with depression if one was afflicted, which is simply not the case.

What we have in some people is a genetic vulnerability that increases the risk of becoming depressed should environmental conditions develop that promote depression. The interplay of genetic and environmental factors needs to be clarified by further research.

In reviewing family and twin studies, as well as studies of depressed persons who have been adopted, the cumulative evidence points to the role that heredity plays in some forms of depression. At this point, the

---

[3]*These figures are based on Allen's (1976) compilation of research. The samples studied are not large and the figures should be considered as rough estimates.*

influence of heredity seems particularly clear and significant for bipolar disorder. The influence of heredity seems less clear and is probably less important for the milder, chronic form of unipolar depression, dysthymic disorder.[4]

New procedures developed in molecular genetics technology are being applied in the search for the specific genes that are involved in the transmission of bipolar disorder. Some initial discoveries have excited researchers: it looks like specific genes implicated in bipolar disorders can be identified. Linkages have been reported between markers on two different chromosomes (chromosome 11 and the X chromosome) and bipolar disorder.[5] There is a road of sophisticated research that remains to be traveled before the genetic mechanisms involved in bipolar disorder are fully clarified, but the advances in molecular genetics technology provide scientists with tools for attacking this problem.

The Neurotransmitters

The search for biological bases for depression has opened up another rich vein of ore in the study of the action of the neurotransmitters. To appreciate the important role neurotransmitters play in our functioning, keep in mind that there are billions of nerve cells (neurons) in the brain. These nerve cells are separated by small gaps called *synapses.* Electrical messages transmitting signals within the brain and relaying instructions to various parts of the body cross these gaps through the action of certain chemicals. When nerve cells release these chemicals, they seep across the gaps to a receptor in an adjacent nerve cell, transmitting the message to "fire" or "not fire." These chemicals are called *neurotransmitters.*

Researchers have identified over a score of neurotransmitters and anticipate finding more. Some of these neurotransmitters, particularly *norepinephrine* and *serotonin,* appear to play a role in depression.

Norepinephrine, also known as *noradrenaline,* may be more familiar

---

[4]*A discussion of hereditary influence in different types of depression is presented in Blehar et al. (1988).*

[5]*See Baron et al. (1987), and Egeland et al. (1987). For a discussion of some of the technical issues involved in linkage studies see Merikangas et al. (1989). In the workshop report, it was indicated that three groups of investigators working in different parts of the world had found evidence for a linkage between X chromosome markers and bipolar disorder.*

in its role in the transmission of impulses in the body's sympathetic nervous system, which prepares the body to react to emergencies. You know the feeling, the "fight or flight" reaction. Your heart rate increases and you begin to sweat. Norepinephrine is also synthesized within the brain and used in the transmission of messages within the brain. So norepinephrine has a dual capacity in the transmission of messages both within and without the brain.

Serotonin is synthesized within the brain. The nerve tracks that use serotonin as a major transmitter are believed to involve the regulation of sleep, hunger, sensitivity to pain and body temperature. The cell bodies of these nerve tracts are located within the brain stem with terminals in the brain and spinal cord.

Researchers have discovered that in many depressed people there are problems in the way these neurotransmitters are working. It may be that there is a faulty synthesis of the chemicals, or the chemicals are not broken down correctly. There are studies showing too little of these substances in the central synapses and other studies showing too much activity. What seems to be the case is that many depressed people have imbalances in norepinephrine and serotonin.

Because the networks that conduct norepinephrine and serotonin penetrate many areas of the brain, sending messages to the centers controlling sleep, appetite and sexual feelings, disturbances in the functions of these neurotransmitters can have widespread effects. And this is exactly what we see in depression, which is a constellation of many symptoms.

One of the interesting findings concerning serotonin is a link to suicide. Autopsies of suicide victims have revealed low levels of serotonin activity, particularly when the victim's suicide was a violent act.[6]

A promising lead for possibly modifying serotonin levels in the brain comes from research carried out by neuroendocrinologist Richard Wurtman. Wurtman and his collaborators found that an amino acid called *tryptophan* controls the amount of serotonin the brain produces. They found that injecting tryptophan solution into laboratory animals increased the level of brain serotonin. What is particularly intriguing is that they also found that diet influences the production of tryptophan. A diet both

[6]*See Mann et al. (1986). The investigators reported an increase in the number of serotonin binding sites in the frontal cortices of violent suicide victims.*

rich in carbohydrates and poor in proteins seems to increase brain serotonin. It is possible that when the role of diet and serotonin is fully clarified, food supplements or special diets will be recommended as an adjunct to the treatment of depression.[7]

At this point, the dynamics of these abnormalities in the neurotransmitters in depressed people are not fully understood. Some researchers have questioned whether the abnormalities are simply a matter of too high or too low an activity level. They have raised the question of whether these neurotransmitters are regulated correctly, suggesting that these systems may be out of kilter. It would be something like if the thermostat in your house or automobile was malfunctioning.

Researchers have used the term *dysregulation* to describe some of the abnormalities observed in these biological systems. In elucidating the concept of dysregulation, Larry Siever and Kenneth Davis discuss such ideas as impaired mechanisms, erratic output, disruption in normal periodicities, less selective response to environmental stimuli, and slower return to basal levels. These ideas conjure up an image of an engine that is out of sync.

The out-of-sync model receives some support from studies of the system producing norepinephrine—the noradrenergic system. According to some reports, the output of this system is more erratic (variable) in depressed patients than normal subjects. There is also evidence that, in some cases, the output on the system shows more fluctuation when a patient is in a depressive episode than when the depressive symptoms have abated. These observations lend credibility to the dysregulation theory.

A Possible Biological Test for Depression

Plasma norepinephrine is stress sensitive. If you should place your hand in ice water and hold it there, you would find it a very unpleasant sensation. This uncomfortable action, which is called "the cold pressor test" is very likely to increase plasma norepinephrine. The same thing would probably happen if someone administered a series of mild electric

---

[7] *The use of tryptophan as a diet supplement has been associated with severe medical problems, including fatalities, probably caused by contamination. It would seem prudent to use the substance only under medical supervision.*

shocks to you. It has been reported that even the act of doing mental arithmetic will cause an increase in plasma norepinephrine.

One noteworthy characteristic of norepinephrine is that it triggers a process that leads to the secretion of the hormone *cortisol*. The process involves the actions of the hypothalamus in the brain and the pituitary and adrenal glands—the *HPA* axis. Cortisol is a stress responsive hormone and appears to be sensitive to depression as well. In a large number of depressed patients, perhaps as many as 60 percent, one finds evidence of hypersecretion of cortisol. Researchers have attempted to capitalize on this observation to develop a test that would be a biological marker for depression. A procedure that has generated a lot of interest is called the *Dexamethasone Suppression Test (DST)*.

For most people, the chemical dexamethasone suppresses the secretion of cortisol for a period of at least 24 hours. Under the influence of this agent, plasma levels of cortisol measured by standardized laboratory procedures are low. While this suppressive effect is found in most normal people, it is not found in many people who are depressed. In many depressed patients, cortisol levels continue to remain high even after taking dexamethasone. The failure to suppress cortisol, then, could be an indication for depression.

The typical procedure for the DST is as follows: 1.0 mg. of dexamethasone is taken at 11:00 P.M. During the following morning, afternoon and evening, blood samples are taken from the patient to check the level of plasma cortisol concentration. An elevation of cortisol in any of the blood samples indicates a failure of the expected suppression activity of the drug, and is considered a positive test result.

How accurately will positive results on the DST identify persons with diagnoses of major depression? After several thousand people had been tested, the provisional answer to this question is that the test picks out about half (45 percent) of individuals with major depression. About one out of ten normal subjects also test positively on the DST.[8]

You can see from these figures that the DST is not as accurate as one would like as a technique for identifying persons with major depression. It would be something like a lie detector test that could pick out people who actually lied about half of the time, although it was reasonably good at clearing people who were telling the truth.

---

[8]*For a review of the DST as a tool in the diagnosis of depression, see the report of the APA Task Force on Laboratory Tests in Psychiatry (1987).*

With the evidence mounting that the DST is not a definitive biological marker for depression, researchers have looked for other possibilities. The abnormalities in the HPA axis observed in many depressed patients still seem like a good bet for further study and there are alternative ways of looking at these abnormalities.

Two such neuroendocrine tests are arginine vasopressin challenge and insulin-induced hypoglycemia. Arginine vasopressin stimulates cortisol secretion; depressed patients tend to exhibit a larger cortisol response to such stimulation than normal subjects. Insulin-induced hypoglycemia tends to affect ACTH levels differently for depressed and normal subjects; depressed patients may show a blunted ACTH response.

Using these endocrine tests, a research team led by William Meller has been able to find more HPA axis abnormalities in depressed cases than they would have simply using the DST alone. Still employing all three tests of HPA axis activity, the researchers were able to find such abnormalities in only a slight majority of depressed patients. The tentative conclusion is that some patients with major depression simply do not have HPA axis abnormalities. The questions then become What does it mean when patients evidence such abnormalities? and What does it mean when they don't? What are the implications for treatment of and recovery from depression?

The DST provides a convenient opportunity to explore these issues. One question that has been asked is, Can the DST pick out those patients who are likely to respond best to antidepressive medications? Studies to date indicate the answer is negative. Suppressors and nonsuppressors respond about equally well to these medications.

A second question followed from the observation that in the course of treatment for depression, some patients change from nonsuppressors of cortisol to suppressors, i.e., DST responses change from positive to negative. Other patients remain DST positive throughout therapy. A comparison of these two groups of patients points to an interesting pattern.

The patient whose DST tests remain positive do not do as well after treatment is completed. They seem more likely to experience serious emotional problems, including suicide attempts, and more often need rehospitalization. This observation suggests that the DST could prove useful in identifying patients who might need increased follow-up care after the initial depressive episode has abated.

Depression and Sleep Patterns

We know that difficulty in sleeping is one of the more common symptoms of depression. Apart from the fact that people who are depressed have trouble falling asleep and may wake up frequently, there are physiological differences in the sleep patterns that distinguish depressed and nondepressed individuals. These differences have been identified in sleep laboratories.

Sleep laboratories were developed as controlled scientific settings to monitor sleep and dream activity. While subjects sleep, their breathing and heart rate are monitored, their brain waves are recorded by an electroencephalograph (EEG), and the movements of their eyes that take place during sleep are recorded with the aid of electrodes pasted on the scalp.

Using this equipment, researchers are able to monitor the various phases of sleep, including the periods of jerky rapid eye movements (REM) during which dreams are most likely to occur.[9]

When persons diagnosed as having a major depression are compared with nondepressed controls in terms of these instrument recordings, a number of differences emerge. For example, there are periods in the sleep cycle in which the EEG pens mark out a pattern of slow, high amplitude waves.

This slow wave sleep, called delta sleep, is usually characterized by deep sleep. When people are experiencing depression, they tend to get less delta sleep than nondepressed controls.

Differences have also been observed for REM sleep. One of the findings that has been reported is that depressed patients tend to have shorter intervals of time (latencies) before they experience rapid eye movements. REM activity seems to be concentrated in the first half of the night. Moreover, severity of depression has been associated with REM density.

In a paper reviewing these and other findings on sleep research, Cindy Ehlers, Ellen Frank and David Kupfer point out that about 90 percent of patients with major depression have at least one indicator of sleep abnormality. They suggest that these disruptions in sleep rhythms could be an important clue in the understanding of depression.

These researchers also look at depression as a state in which there is

---

[9]*For a detailed description of REM research, see Robbins (1988), chapter 3.*

a dysregulation or disruption of certain biological processes. These processes include both the neuroendocrine system, which we have already discussed, and the sleep-wake cycle. In the latter instance, it is as if one's biological clock is out of kilter, something like a case of perpetual jet lag. There is a possible tie-in of this view to one type of depression—seasonal depression, the depressed state that typically sets in during winter, abates in spring and responds to treatment with bright artificial light. It may be that the bright light acts to synchronize rhythms that have become disrupted.

Extending the theory of dysregulation into the realm of social interaction, Ehlers and her colleagues note that environmental events can affect biological rhythms. They point to the commonplace observation of how one's sleeping and eating habits are affected by living with others. Think of life before and after marriage. The authors mention the interesting research that found that the depressive effects of bereavement were less evident in widows who maintained the usual routines of daily life as much as possible.

The biological desynchronization that takes place in depression and the influence of social and environmental causes in producing this condition are important ideas to keep in mind as we pursue our inquiries in subsequent chapters, particularly when we consider the effects of stress in triggering depressive reactions.

We know from much research that REM sleep is associated with dreaming, and we also know that the REM patterns of persons with major depression are atypical. These observations raise questions about the dreams of people who are depressed—what are they like?

My own research carried out on normal subjects indicates that when people are in a depressed mood, they tend to have better dream recall than when their mood is more positive. This better recall may simply reflect a tendency for people not to sleep as well when they are troubled; nocturnal awakenings help one remember one's dreams. In contrast to normal subjects, people who are very depressed tend to have rather poor dream recall. Their dreams are usually short and banal. During the height of depression, recall for dreams, many of which can arouse uncomfortable feelings, seems to be at a low point. There may be some kind of psychological or biological mechanism operating to reduce stress.

A final note about sleep. Depressed mood is sometimes associated with sleep-related respiratory disturbance, a condition characterized by loud and disruptive snoring. In the sleep laboratory, researchers have found that in elderly males, this sleep respiratory problem was associated with depressed mood.[10]

Depression and the Immune System

We have noticed that when people feel depressed, they are more likely to experience stress-related physical complaints such as headaches, dizziness, nausea and diarrhea. Moreover, there are reports that when people are clinically depressed, they have higher rates of infections, autoimmune and neoplastic diseases.[11] These observations have led researchers to ask the question: Does depression lower the body's resistance to fighting off disease? And more specifically, is there a relation between depression and the functioning of the body's immune system?

Because of inconsistencies in research findings, one must be cautious about drawing conclusions about these questions. There is evidence pointing to a possible association between depression and measures of immune system functioning.[12] In some studies, it has been observed that depressed people have decreased numbers of T-cells. Some researchers have reported lower numbers of both helper and suppressor T-cells. One of the most interesting findings is a report of an inverse relation between the extent to which people are depressed as measured by psychological tests and their T-cell counts: the higher the score on depression, the lower the T-cell count.

What happens when depressed symptoms clear up, when depression is in a state of remission? Does the activity of the immune system appear normal? There is some evidence that this may be the case. When researchers studied depressed people whose symptoms had remitted, and compared them with normal controls, they found no difference in T-cell counts. The relation of depression and the immune system is an important, unsettled problem requiring further study.

In these thumbnail sketches, I have tried to show that depression is not only a psychological or behavioral disorder, but has both biological causes and biological consequences. One can envision a time when testing for biological abnormalities might become a routine part of the

[10]*See Bliwise et al. (1986).*
[11]*See Denney et al. (1988) for a review of these studies.*
[12]*See Denney et al. (1988).*

diagnostic workup for patients experiencing severe depression. Clinical neuroscience programs already in place in some psychiatric hospitals are being used in the evaluation of depressed patients. These programs offer such services as magnetic resonance imaging and EEG studies during sleep. It seems likely that additional tests will be developed, based on the kinds of research discussed in this chapter, that will assist the mental health professional in better understanding his or her depressed patients.

BIBLIOGRAPHY

Allen, M. G. (1976). Twin studies of affective illness. *Archives of General Psychiatry*, 33, 1476–78.

The APA Task Force on Laboratory Tests in Psychiatry (1987). The Dexamethasone Suppression Test: An overview of its current status in psychiatry. *American Journal of Psychiatry*, 144, 1253–62.

Baron, M.; Risch, N.; Hamburger, R.; Mandel, B.; Kushner, S.; Newman, M.; Drumer, D.; & Belmaker, R. (1987). Genetic linkage between X-chromosome markers and affective illness. *Nature*, 326, 289–92.

Blehar, M. C.; Weissman, M. M.; Gershon, E. S.; & Hirschfeld, R. M. A. (1988). Family and genetic studies of affective disorders. *Archives of General Psychiatry*, 45, 289–92.

Bliwise, D. L.; Yesavage, J. A.; Sink, J.; Windrow, L.; & Dement, W. C. (1986). Depressive symptoms and impaired respiration in sleep. *Journal of Consulting and Clinical Psychology*, 54, 734–35.

Brantley, P. J.; Dietz, L. S.; McKnight, G. T.; Jones, G. N.; & Tulley, R. (1988). Convergence between the daily stress inventory and endocrine measures of stress. *Journal of Consulting and Clinical Psychology*, 56, 549–51.

Chollar, S. (1988, April). Food for thought. *Psychology Today*, 22, 30–34.

Denney, D. R.; Stephenson, L. A.; Penick, E. C.; & Weller, R. A. (1988). Lymphocyte subclass and depression. *Journal of Abnormal Psychology*, 97, 499–502.

Egeland, J. A.; Gerhard, D. S.; Pauls, D. L.; Sussex, J. N.; Kidd, K. K.; Allen, C. R.; Hostetter, A. M.; & Houseman, D. A. (1987). Bipolar affective disorders linked to DNA markers on chromosome 11. *Nature*, 325, 783–87.

Ehlers, C. L.; Frank, E.; & Kupfer, D. J. (1988). Social zeitgebers and biological rhythms. *Archives of General Psychiatry*, 45, 948–52.

Flaherty, J.; Frank, E.; Hoskinson, K.; Richman, J.; & Kupfer, D. (1987, May). Social zeitgebers and bereavement. Paper presented American Psychiatric Association, Chicago.

Gallagher, W. C. (1986, May). The dark affliction of mind and body. *Discover*, 7, no. 5, 66–76.

Kendler, K. S.; Heath, A.; Martin, N. G.; & Eaves, L. J. (1986). Symptoms of anxiety and depression in a volunteer twin population. *Archives of General Psychiatry*, 43, 213–21.

Mann, J. J.; Stanley, M.; McBride, P. A.; & McEwen, B. S. (1986). Increased serotonin and B-adrenergic receptor binding in the frontal cortices of suicide victims. *Archives of General Psychiatry*, 43, 954–59.

Meller, W.; Kathol, R. G.; Jaeckle, R. S.; Grambsch, P.; & Lopez, J. F. (1988). HPA axis abnormalities in depressed patients with normal response to the DST. *American Journal of Psychiatry*, 145, 318–24.

Merikangas, K. R.; Spence, A. M.; & Kupfer, D. J. (1989). Linkage studies of bipolar disorder: Methodologic and analytic issues. Report of MacArthur Foundation Workshop on Linkage and Clinical Features in Affective Disorders. *Archives of General Psychology*, 46, 1137–41.

Robbins, P. R. (1988). *The Psychology of Dreams*. Jefferson, N.C.: McFarland.
_____, & Tanck, R. H. (1988). Depressed mood, dream recall and content-less dreams. *Imagination, Cognition and Personality*, 8, 165–74.

Sargent, M. (1986). *Depressive disorders: Treatments bring new hope*. DHHS publication no. (ADM) 86-1491.

Siever, L. J., & Davis, K. L. (1985). Overview: Toward a dysregulation hypothesis of depression. *American Journal of Psychiatry*, 142, 1017–31.

Weisman, R. (1984, March). Nutrition and neurotransmitters: The research of Richard Wurtman. *NIMH Science Reporter*, 1–8.

Wurtman, R. J. (1982). Nutrients that modify brain function. *Scientific American*, 246, 50–59.

4. A Psychological Perspective on Depression

People who feel depressed tend to have different views of themselves and the world about them than people who are not depressed. These differences have been identified by clinical observation of depressed patients and confirmed by subsequent research. Some theorists like Aaron Beck have proposed that these beliefs or thought patterns play a large role in bringing on depressed mood, assuming that these thought patterns give rise to the sadness experienced in depression.[1]

This theory is an interesting one because it leads to the idea that if you can change thinking patterns, you may be able to alter depressed states. This is the basis for *cognitive therapy* for depression (the word *cognitive* coming from cognitions or ideas). In cognitive therapy, the therapist tries to help the patient change his or her depressive beliefs. The good news is that many studies have found this approach is helpful.

How do the world and the self look to the person who has become depressed? As a way of beginning our discussion, let's consider three people whose moods have recently become depressed. Debbie is a housewife. She stays at home and looks after two school-aged children. Her husband, Tom, works long hours at his job and is usually tired when he comes home. Tom is a good provider, nice with the children when he has the time, quiet spoken, never abusive—but he doesn't give Debbie

---

[1] *While Beck viewed "the negative processing of information" as primary, in that it leads to the other symptoms of depression, he does not view negative thoughts as the cause of depression. In reviewing the status of cognitive therapy, he wrote, "it seems far-fetched to assign a causal role to cognitions because the negative automatic thoughts constitute an integral part of depression, just like the motivational, affective, and behavioral symptoms. To conclude that cognitions cause depression is analogous to asserting that delusions cause schizophrenia." Beck (1991), 373, 369.*

the attention she feels she needs. She feels the spark has gone out of their marriage. The romance of courtship and the early days of marriage seem like a distant memory. Now her life seems like an endless series of chores—shopping, cooking, cleaning, chauffeuring. She feels people expect things from her all the time and she feels little sense of accomplishment or fulfillment. More and more she feels trapped. Lately, she's taken to watching soap operas and fantasizing about having affairs. But the idea leaves her very uncomfortable and it remains only a fantasy. She has been drinking a lot and sleeping badly. Occasionally she "blows up," giving some hint of the resentment that has been building. Most of the time, however, she just goes through the motions. When her best friend asked her what was wrong, she only replied, "What's the use?"

Alan is a 20-year-old sophomore student at a suburban community college. His mood plummeted after his first day of class in economics. During the class, the professor had outlined what she was planning to cover in the course. When the class was over, Alan sat down on a bench on the campus and pictured in his mind what lay ahead. The course outline sounded difficult. He didn't understand some of the things the professor had said. The student in the class who asked questions seemed very sharp. Alan wondered whether he could compete. During the previous semester he had had a bad experience in a math class, and didn't economics involve math? Maybe the best thing was not to take the risk. Better to drop the course than fail again. Alan felt a sense of defeat, a sense of giving up that he had experienced before.

Linda is a teacher in the seventh grade in a large metropolitan area. When she first started teaching four years ago, she did so enthusiastically, feeling a real calling for teaching and a desire to make a difference in the lives of the children. She was quite unprepared for all of the problems she ran into. Some of the students had behavior problems: they were unruly and seemed to delight in disrupting the class. Many of the students were unprepared for the work and seemed unmotivated to learn. Truancy was a repeated problem. Some students were using and selling drugs. The school had been vandalized several times, windows had been broken and there had been serious episodes of violence in the corridors.

Linda found it was very hard to create a classroom atmosphere that enabled her to teach and the students to learn. Many of her colleagues reported the same problem. The school principal knew this but felt helpless to do very much about it.

Linda liked many of her students and she had good friends on the staff. Still, she had become demoralized. She had no idea of what she could do to change things at the school. If the school administration couldn't do anything, what chance did she have? Increasingly she began to dread going to work and longed for the weekends. On Sunday nights she felt panicky and had trouble sleeping. In her eyes, the school situation had become a perpetual bad dream.

There is a pattern running through these cases. In each instance, the individual looks at her or his situation in life in a negative way and feels pessimistic about the possibility of change. The outlook boils down to this: "My situation is bad and I cannot do anything to make things better." A tendency to view one's situation in a negative way and a feeling of powerlessness to do anything about it are cornerstones of a depression-related mind-set.

The Negative Perspective

When we talk about having a negative perspective, we are talking about a tendency to view events in a negative rather than positive light. It is a mind-set in which you evaluate yourself and the world you live in unfavorably. Consider the proverbial glass that may be seen as half full or half empty; the negative perspective views it as half empty.

Aaron Beck, who has been one of the principal architects of the negative thinking pattern approach to depression, sees this negative perspective applying to one's view of oneself, the world about one and the future. It's a "triple whammy." In therapy, we often listen to patients describe their lives as unpleasant. They may relate grim details about their job and find little appealing in their home lives. Their worlds appear unpromising and unrewarding.

Now, there may be a good deal of truth in what the depressed person points out. In therapy, the patient may complain, "I'm not getting anywhere in life," and this may be true. The job situation and home life may present real problems. However, depressed people, like everyone else, have a tendency towards *selective perception.* To varying degrees, people see what they want to see and hear what they want to hear. It is something like what happens during a political campaign. You may listen to a candidate on a television program who says things you agree with, but turn off one who says things you disagree with. The depressed person may present a reasonably accurate picture as far as it goes, but it is likely to be selective. He or she may be ignoring things that could make the overall picture seem a good deal brighter than it appears.

While some persons with tendencies toward depression engage in bouts of self-analysis and reason themselves into negative conclusions, negative thinking processes often have an almost automatic character. Such thoughts seem to chase across the depressed person's stream of consciousness something like the spots or floaters that chase across people's eyes when a section of vitreous in the eye becomes detached. At times, these depressive thought patterns have an almost obsessive quality.

In his book *Cognitive Therapy and the Emotional Disorders,* Aaron Beck related how he first became sensitized to these automatic thoughts while he was doing psychoanalytic therapy. When he became convinced of the importance of these automatic thoughts, he began to ask his patients to pay particular attention to them and to report them to him. He told his patients that when they experienced unpleasant feelings, to try to recall the thoughts they had prior to the feelings.[2]

Beck observed that automatic thoughts were typically discrete and specific, resembling a kind of shorthand. The patients did not try to initiate the thoughts; they simply occurred. Once the thought appeared in the patient's consciousness, it was hard for the patient to get rid of it. These thoughts could not be easily turned off like water from a faucet.

Beck reported that while outside observers might consider the negative ideas of depressed patients to be farfetched, the patients felt they were reasonable and true. In talking with a patient, one might be able to persuade her or him that these thoughts didn't make a lot of sense, but in a short period of time, the patient might soon revert to believing the ideas as strongly as ever. The negative thoughts that may preoccupy the mind of a depression-prone person can be resilient.

The tendency for depressed people to view their own performance negatively has been demonstrated in experiments. For example, in one study, depressed and nondepressed subjects took part in an individualized learning experiment. The subjects had to learn to associate particular numbers with particular words. Each time the subject responded, the experimenter would say whether she or he was right or wrong. At a point in the learning experiment, the researchers asked the subjects to

---

[2]*Beck (1976), p. 33.*

estimate what percentage of their prior responses were correct. The depressed subjects were more likely to *underestimate* how often they had been told they were correct than the nondepressed subjects.[3]

There is an increasing body of research that suggests that the negative evaluations of depressed people are only part of the equation. People who are not depressed may have a tendency to *inflate* how well they have performed in experimental studies.[4] People who are not depressed may have some degree of illusion about their performance. As we shall speculate later, this positive, optimistic perspective may act as a kind of protective shield against depressive reactions.

Powerlessness

Powerlessness is a belief that you are at the mercy of external events and there is little or nothing you can do to change things. Like negative thought patterns, feeling powerless is associated with depression.

Researchers have studied one aspect of the relation of powerlessness and depression at length, and that is the extent to which people view the sources of gratification in their life as being under the control of external forces or under their own control. The hypothesis is that the former (external) view would be associated with depression. In testing this idea, researchers have used psychological tests to measure a person's perception of internal vs. external control. How might such a test look? Suppose someone presented you with pairs of items like "getting somewhere in life is a matter of hard work," and "the most important thing about achieving success is being lucky," and asked you to check the item that is closer to your way of thinking. If you checked many items like the second, you would receive a high external score.[5]

After examining studies exploring the relation between perceived locus of control and measures of depression, Victor Benassi and his colleagues concluded, "We found strong support for the hypothesis that greater externality is associated with greater depression."[6]

One facet of powerlessness is a belief that the world you live in is

[3]*See Buchwald (1977).*
[4]*For example, Lewinsohn et al. (1980).*
[5]*A scale widely used to measure the perception of control of reinforcement was developed by Julian Rotter. See Rotter (1960).*
[6]*Benassi et al. (1988), p. 362.*

composed of immovable obstacles that will prove resistant to anything you try to do. No matter what you try to do, the result will be something like running into a stone wall. The outcome of such a view is likely to be, "I won't be able to do anything, so what's the use of trying." Martin Seligman has referred to reactions like this as *learned helplessness.* The idea is that your experiences have led you to conclude that your own efforts have no clear effect on outcomes and events. Life appears something like a slot machine—a one-armed bandit that doesn't pay off.[7]

The belief that what you do is not going to make any difference is something that may be learned from repeated frustrations. The phenomenon has been demonstrated in experiments. Here is an example: The subject is exposed to an unpleasant condition like loud noise. The subject presses a button in an attempt to turn the noise off, but finds that pushing the button doesn't stop the noise. The subject gives up. When put into a similar situation where pushing a new device (a knob) would actually turn off the noise, the subject is less likely to even try it. He may sit passively and remain uncomfortable while the noise blasts away.[8]

Perhaps an even more debilitating form of powerlessness than believing that the environment is stacked against you is the feeling that you are incompetent and can't do anything. Believing the environment is the problem at least offers some protection for your self-esteem. Believing that you are incompetent doesn't leave you many "outs" psychologically.

Feelings of inadequacy—the idea that "I can't do it" or "I won't measure up"—are another form of learned helplessness. This belief typically has its roots in childhood, in frustrating, unsuccessful experiences, and in disparaging messages communicated from parents, peers and teachers. Repeated experiences of nonrewarded performance and derision erode self-confidence and lead to the conclusion, "I'm not capable."

Janet Altman and J. R. Wittenborn gave out questionnaires to a group of women who had once experienced a serious depression and to a group of nondepressed controls. There were consistent differences between the groups in reported confidence, perceived competence and self-esteem. The women who had been depressed were more likely to

---

[7]*For a review of research on learned helplessness, see the special February 1978 issue of the* Journal of Abnormal Psychology, *entitled "Learned Helplessness as a Model of Depression."*

[8]*See Hiroto (1974).*

respond that it was hard to credit themselves with good, doubted that they deserved praise, were uncomfortable with responsibility, often failed unnecessarily, and were not good enough to try for the top.

The consequence of learned helplessness and feelings of powerlessness are likely to include a passive life-style. A person is less likely to take risks when the thought of failure looms large and is more willing to tolerate an unpleasant state of affairs—a cramped and limited life-style if it seems secure. The chances are higher that he or she may fall into a dependency relationship with someone perceived as more competent.

The tendency to view oneself and one's environment in a negative way, in conjunction with a perception that one is powerless to change things, may ultimately lead to a feeling of hopelessness, that one is boxed into a miserable life. Things haven't worked out well to date, and there's no prospect that they ever will. When problems seem insolvable and when a feeling of hopelessness becomes lodged in one's consciousness, suicidal thoughts may develop. The playwright Jean Anouilh described the feeling aptly in his play *Restless Heart* when he spoke of "the farthest limits of his pain" and "the far end of despair."[9]

The feeling of hopelessness casts a bleak shadow over one's daily experience. The depressed person often feels that time lingers, that the day is interminable. If put to a test of estimating how much time has actually elapsed between two settings on the clock, people who are in a depressed mood are likely to do as well as anyone else—it is the subjective evaluation of experience that is different.[10] Life seems to have little movement and vitality. It is as if the depressed person is cast in a mental prison.

A person looking from the outside with a more objective perspective can see that this mental prison is often not a true assessment of the way things are or could be. Except for a terminal illness for which all remedies have been exhausted, there are very few things in life that are hopeless. Separation or divorce is an antidote to a very bad marriage. One can change jobs. Joining a club is a step toward ending loneliness. Few bad situations are unalterable. But the depressed person has to alter his view to see that this mental prison is more apparent than real and that some things can be done.

[9]*Anouilh (1959), Act 3, p. 64.*
[10]*See Hawkins et al. (1988).*

Some Depressive Thought Patterns

Let's turn our attention to some of the thought patterns often found in depressed people that contribute to the feeling of hopelessness. One of these patterns is a tendency to overgeneralize. It is the classic case of $2+2=5$, or perhaps even 50.

Take Liz, who works in a large office in an insurance company. Every week Liz has contacts with about 20 other employees. One of these employees, Barbara, had a nasty argument with Liz and now walks right past Liz without speaking to her. Another woman, Judy, is also unfriendly to Liz, but Judy is unfriendly to just about everyone in the office. What has Liz concluded? That no one likes her at the office—and worse, that she is unlikeable. One could point out to Liz that if she listed all of the people in the office, and went through the names one by one, she would find there were many people in her office who are in fact friendly to her. But Liz, like many people who become depressed, has overgeneralized from a few incidents and drawn a sweeping conclusion.

Overgeneralization may take the form that if some things are wrong in life, then everything is wrong. And if things are bad in the foreseeable future, they will always be bad. Overgeneralization in depressed people has been demonstrated in psychological experiments. For example, in an experiment in which the subjects had been told they had done poorly in a "social perceptiveness test," the subjects who were more depressed tended to magnify and overgeneralize their failure. As the authors Richard Wenzlaff and Sherilyn Grozier describe their results, "the failure feedback had more far-reaching effects on depressed subjects' self-perceptions than on those of nondepressed subjects. After learning they had done poorly on a test of social perceptiveness, depressed subjects not only lowered their estimates of their social perceptiveness, but also believed they were generally less proficient."[11] The subjects also tended to magnify the importance of what they had been tested on.

Along the same lines, Charles Carver and Ronald Ganellen developed a questionnaire measure of the tendency to overgeneralize, using such items as, "When even one thing goes wrong I begin to feel bad and wonder if I can do well at anything at all," and "How I feel about myself overall is easily influenced by a single mistake."[12] The researchers

[11] *Wenzlaff & Grozier (1988), p. 93.*
[12] *Carver & Ganellen (1983), p. 333.*

found that people who scored high on this measure were more likely to score high on a measure of depression.

Perfectionism and black and white categorization are other forms of thinking that may contribute to depression. When one hears the phrase "he's a perfectionist," one thinks of a person who has a very high level of aspiration. His goals are not only high, they may be out of sight. He may pay inordinate attention to details, imposing exacting standards that everything must be "just so." If it isn't right, you do it again. There is an obsessive striving to attain a standard that may not be reachable. What might be seen as reasonable progress by another person may be seen only as failure.

An example of problems that come with perfectionist thinking is the student who is hung up on grades. If only an A grade will do and she doesn't get an A, where is she? Disappointed, maybe depressed.

In therapy, I have often heard statements like "My father said, if you can't do it right, don't do it at all." This overly demanding standard didn't help the people who consulted me and I wonder how much good it did for their fathers and mothers. If the only standard one can accept is perfection, then who can possibly meet it? The consequence of perfectionist thinking is often not being happy with what you do or not being willing to try anything because of the belief it may not turn out good enough. Both of these tendencies can contribute to a depressed mood.

Black and white categorization is a tendency to evaluate things in an extreme way—as being either "super" or "lousy"—and to not see what is in between. One often finds some intolerance with this perspective, a predilection to classify people as wonderful or terrible and not as the mix of strengths and frailties that they really are. With this outlook, one can come down very hard on people—and pretty soon one may find oneself with few friends. Being without friends often translates into feeling lonely, which in turn may translate into depressed mood.

Albert Ellis, writing from the perspective of rational-emotive therapy, has developed a list of "irrational beliefs" that are related to depression. Ellis includes such beliefs as a need to excel in everything one does to feel worthwhile as a person, the idea that it is *terrible* when things are not going the way one would like them to go, and that one cannot overcome the effects of past history.[13] Aaron Beck has developed a similar sounding list of attitudes that he believes predisposes people to sadness

[13]*See Ellis, A. (1962).*

or depression. These attitudes contain elements of perfectionist and absolutist thinking, as well as a tendency to view events in one's life as being under external control.[14]

As these researchers suggest, many depression-prone people apply excessively demanding standards to themselves. Freud would have talked about a demanding superego. Imagine that your life is being run by a permanent drill sergeant who tolerates no excuses, sees no extenuating circumstances and sees no shades of gray in life. With this mental makeup, it's not a big step to arrive at a conclusion that one has fallen short of almost everything and to find one's self-esteem deflated.

People can further tear down their self-esteem and drive themselves deeper into the mental prison of depression by frequently comparing themselves with others who seem to be doing better. Comparing oneself with others on occasion is not unusual, but many depressed people have a habit of doing this, and they do so in a way that deepens their feelings of inadequacy. The comparisons emphasize their shortcomings, not their strong points. If you think about it, you can always find someone who seems smarter or better looking, or makes more money or has nicer furniture, or is a better athlete, or whatever else is important to you. Measuring oneself by the accomplishments (or perceived accomplishments) of others can leave one chronically frustrated and discontented.

Many people who become depressed spend a lot of time thinking about themselves. Attention is focused inwardly rather than on things to do in the external world. While occasional self-monitoring can be a good thing, it is not usually helpful to make a career out of it. Moreover, the problem is compounded by the tendency of depressed people to have a negative bias in their thinking. Excessive inward attention may simply be *multiplying negatives.* Constantly turning over the question of "What's wrong with me?" is unlikely to make a person feel positive about anything.

Resentment and Anger

When we accumulate these psychological patterns—a focus on the negative, a feeling of powerlessness, overgeneralization, perfectionist thinking, and the tendency to come down hard on oneself—one can see

[14]*Beck (1976), p. 255.*

why self-esteem takes a beating and mood is likely to plummet. The person may become paralyzed in this mental prison and rendered inactive and ineffectual. He or she may also become angry.

Anger sometimes takes the form of a deep sense of resentment. We are talking about people who may become frustrated by what is happening in their lives. They may be frustrated by not being able to do what they want, or their view of reality may be so negatively skewed that they are not able to enjoy what they are accomplishing. When this happens, the person may feel like a "victim," looking at the world about her or him as unfair. Developing resentment may be directed against one's family and friends, or turned inwardly against oneself.

In psychoanalytic theory, the concept of anger turned inward occupies a central place in the causation of depression. The idea has its roots in a seminal essay of Sigmund Freud's entitled *Mourning and Melancholia.*[15] Freud was struck by some of the similarities between mourning following the death of a loved one and depression. He believed that depression, too, was based upon the experience of loss, but that the dynamics of what happened were more complex. Freud wrote that in depression the relationship between the person who becomes depressed and the lost loved one is not a straightforward positive one; rather, the depressed persons' feelings are characterized by marked ambivalence, that is, the presence of both positive and negative feelings. The negative feelings often arise from incidents in the relationship in which the person was disappointed, hurt and neglected. Freud wrote of an ensuing struggle in the person's unconscious in which feelings of love and hostility wrestle with each other. The struggle resolves itself not by the anger being overtly expressed towards the person who "provoked" it, or by the person giving up his or her love; rather, the anger is displaced, turned inwardly against the self. The person describes him- or herself as worthless, rather than describing the lost loved one, the one who rejected him or her, as such. In this process, a degree of revenge is often exacted as the depressive illness provides a means of tormenting the person who injured the depressed person's feelings.

It is an intriguing scenario, a testament to Freud's ingenuity and remarkable powers of clinical observation. And, indeed, one often sees elements of the scenario in depressed patients, the experience of loss,

---

[15]*This essay, along with theoretical writings by others in the psychoanalytic movement, has generated considerable research on the relation of anger and depression.*

anger and remorse. The patient's resentment toward others, however, may be anything but buried in the unconscious. Resentment may be simmering on the surface, if not boiling. My distinct impression is that anger toward others may coexist with anger toward the self.

When we work with depressed patients, we often see self-reproach as part of the clinical picture. In interpreting this, one must keep in mind the psychoanalytic view that some of these negative feelings toward the self have as their true target someone else. A man might feel very angry about his wife or boss, but may be unable to express these feelings, and eventually this resentment comes home to roost. It is not clear, however, that self-reproach is always an unconscious process of displaced anger. An individual may begin to recognize his own shortcomings and failures in dealing with his problems and react in self-disgust. One can picture a sequence of thoughts, "I can't do it . . . I'm no good . . . Damn it!" Perhaps both conscious and unconscious processes are at work in directing anger inwardly.

If self-directed anger plays a role in the depressive process, we should expect to see less of this as the patient improves in therapy. There is some research that indicates that this is the case.

The Measurement of Mind-Sets

We have discussed a number of mind-sets, attitudes and personality tendencies that seem to promote depressive reactions. Psychologists have been developing instruments to measure the various mind-sets. We have already mentioned questionnaires that assess perceived external vs. internal control of reinforcement and a tendency to overgeneralize. Other self-report measures that have been developed are questionnaires that assess the frequency of automatic thoughts, typical styles for interpreting negative experiences and the tendency to hold irrational beliefs. All of these techniques have been used by researchers in trying to more clearly understand the role of psychological factors in depression.

As an illustration of these techniques, consider the Automatic Thoughts Questionnaire. Imagine a list of very short statements in front of you, such as "My future is bleak," "Something has to change," "I'm a failure," "I wish I were somewhere else," "No one understands me," "I'm so disappointed in myself," and "I feel so helpless." Your instructions are to indicate, on a five-point scale ranging from "not at all" to "all the time," how frequently these thoughts occurred to you over the last week.[16] You can readily see that if you often had such thoughts, you would qualify for a depressive mind-set.

Here is an informal exercise you might want to try. Think back to some of the more stressful or disappointing experiences of recent months and consider the way you interpreted them. For example, think about a disappointment in a romantic relationship or a stressful problem that happened on your job or at school. Take a moment and go over the situation in your mind. What was your reaction like? How did you evaluate the situation?

Did you tend to catastrophize the situation by thinking "My whole life is in shambles" or "Things will never get any better"?

Did you go through a period of time in which you blamed yourself for what happened?

Did you conclude you were not a worthwhile person?

Now go back a little further in time to another incident in which you experienced stress or disappointment. Once again take some time and think about how you felt and what was going through your mind. Ask yourself the same set of questions.

If you answered yes to most of the questions for both incidents, think back to other episodes and ask yourself the questions. Is this typical for you? Is this your characteristic way of reacting to stressful and disappointing situations? If it is, then you could well have the type of mind-set that makes you vulnerable to depression, a concern you may want to address.

Christopher Peterson and Peter Villanova have developed a psychological test called the Attributional Style Questionnaire (ASQ) which uses hypothetical situations rather than real experiences such as we posed in this informal exercise. The ASQ yields scores that can be used by researchers to investigate the role of thought patterns in the development and maintenance of depression.

The psychological factors we have profiled for depression probably don't work in isolation from one another; most likely they augment one another producing a cumulative effect. Perfectionist tendencies, for example, are likely to increase the chances of self-reproach. A description of this in-

[16]*See Hollon & Kendall (1980). The items for the Automatic Thoughts Questionnaire are listed in table 1, p. 389.*

teraction is offered in a theoretical paper by H. A. Meyersburg and his colleagues: ". . . Guilt is often tied to failures in perfectionistic expectations. Perfectionism is absolute, an all-or-nothing issue. Even a slight falling short of the mark is tantamount to total failure. The tighter the perfectionistic system, the greater the sense of inadequacy at failure and the greater the likelihood of triggering the escalating depressogenic process."[17]

Meyersburg and his colleagues believe that in the face of severe stress coming with loss and disappointment, a constellation of psychological factors—impulsivity, perfectionism, guilt and self-punitiveness—interact with one another as a kind of reverberating mechanism, escalating anxiety to the point where it becomes overwhelming. The reverberating mechanism helps to turn a difficult situation into a psychological debacle.

Mind-sets, attitudes and personality tendencies act as a kind of filtering system between the stressors of the world—the things that can go wrong and often do—and our reactions as human beings. These psychological factors play an important role in determining whether a person becomes seriously depressed. While persons with depressive mind-sets have heightened vulnerability, it is important to recognize that attitudes and mind-sets can be *changed* and, as we shall see, this often takes place in therapy.

The Protective Shield

Frustration and disappointments are near universals in life. Even the best job and the most wonderful family will have their share of unpleasant times. And the less than super job that many of us have and the typical family most of us are in will produce problems aplenty. The person who is relatively free from depression seems to have a kind of protective shield against these daily stresses. He or she is able to tolerate frustrations and disappointments without experiencing sustained periods of depressed mood.

While part of what we call a protective shield is biological and genetically based, there are important psychological components as well.

[17]*Meyersburg et al. (1974), p. 376.*

The idea of a protective shield was suggested in part from unexpected findings in psychological experiments carried out with depressed and nondepressed subjects. Following is an example of one of these experiments: Imagine you have been recruited to take part in the study. You were told that "the investigators were interested in learning more about how people who are strangers relate to one another."[18] You find yourself in a room with four or five other people. You don't know that some of the people are being treated for depression at the university psychology clinic.

All of the people in the group are asked to give three-minute introductory statements about themselves. Then everybody makes conversation for another twenty minutes. At the end of the session, you fill out a rating form asking about your perceptions of the behavior of the other people and yourself during the session. The rating form includes a number of positive descriptions, such as friendly, warm, communicates clearly, interested in other people, socially skillful, and so on. While you take part in this conversational exercise, observers watch you and the other participants through one-way vision screens. They can see you; you can't see them. These observers make the same ratings that you do. Three additional sessions are held at later times.

As the researchers expected, the participants who were clinically depressed evaluated their own performance more negatively than the other subjects. What was not expected, however, was that the nondepressed subjects had a more favorable view of their own performance than was given them by the outside observers.

When the depressed patients improved during treatment, they began to rate themselves more favorably than the outside observers did, just like the nondepressed subjects were doing. In speculating about their findings, the researchers, Peter Lewinsohn and his colleagues, stated, "It is tempting to conjecture that a key to avoiding depression is to see oneself less stringently and more favorably than others see one."[19] The authors use such terms as an "illusory glow in their self-perceptions" to describe the nondepressed subjects.[20]

This study, as well a number of other studies with similar results, suggest that one of the ways of resisting the stressors that promote depres-

[18]*Lewinsohn et al. (1980), p. 205.*
[19]*Lewinsohn et al. (1980), p. 212.*
[20]*Lewinsohn et al. (1980) p. 211.*

sion is to have an optimistic, positive attitude, a tendency to put the best face on circumstances and to believe that one can bring events under control.

As an example, consider possible reactions to an unsuccessful undertaking, such as doing badly on a test at school. One could look at one's performance in a very negative way or one could frame the event in such a way as to protect one's self-esteem. These "reframing maneuvers," as C. R. Snyder calls them, make things seem not as bad. As Snyder puts it, they soften, bleach and repackage the act that may generate self-blame and diminish self-esteem.

One may soften the poor mark on the test with explanations such as "Most people would not have done any better," "The test was extremely difficult," "I was preoccupied with others things that were bothering me and couldn't concentrate," "The test really wasn't that important, anyway," or "I wasn't at my best—I'm not a machine." While one can't make a living on perpetual rationalizations, protecting one's ego from a debacle when one experiences failure has the decided advantage of allowing one to pick oneself up and regroup, to try again without going through a protracted malaise.

The concept of a psychological shield protecting a person against the storms of reality is reminiscent of Charles Dickens' character Mr. McCawber, who is able to cope with the most miserable circumstances with an outlook "something is bound to turn up!" The outlook is something like seeing that half full glass, three-quarters full. Or to use the cliché—to look at life through rose-colored glasses.

Such an attitude may be clearly unrealistic at times, but a strong dose of optimism may act as a deflector, bouncing off stressors like force fields repelling attackers in a science fiction story.

This notion of a psychological protective shield bears a resemblance to the concept of the defense mechanisms postulated by psychoanalytic theories. Defense mechanisms act to protect the ego from being overwhelmed.

We are not suggesting that we should all become Pollyannas or dismiss reality. Remember the character Ilya in the movie *Never on Sunday*? When she related the grim story of Medea, she concluded not with the story's horrible blood bath, but with everyone going for an outing to the beach. We are not suggesting that people follow her example. We are, however, suggesting that optimistic thinking has value in warding off depression.

BIBLIOGRAPHY

Altman, J. H., & Wittenborn, J. R. (1980). Depression-prone personality in women. *Journal of Abnormal Psychology,* 89, 303–8.

Anouilh, J. (1959). Restless heart. In *Five Plays,* Volume II. New York: Hill and Wang.

Beck, A. T. (1976). *Cognitive therapy and the emotional disorders.* New York: International University Press.

————. (1991). Cognitive therapy: A 30-year restrospective. *American Psychologist,* 46, 368–75.

Benassi, V. A.; Sweeney, P. D.; & Dufour, C. L. (1988). Is there a relation between locus of control orientation and depression? *Journal of Abnormal Psychology,* 97, 357–67.

Buchwald, A. M. (1977). Depressive mood and estimates of reinforcement frequency. *Journal of Abnormal Psychology,* 86, 443–46.

Carver, C. S., & Ganellen, R. J. (1983). Depression and components of self-punitiveness: High standards, self criticism, and overgeneralization. *Journal of Abnormal Psychology,* 92, 330–37.

Dickens, C. (1981). *David Copperfield.* Oxford: Oxford University Press.

Dobson, K. S. (1989). A meta-analysis of the efficacy of cognitive therapy for depression. *Journal of Consulting and Clinical Psychology,* 57, 414–19.

Ellis, A. (1962). *Reason and emotion in psychotherapy.* New York: Lyle Stuart.

Freud, S. (1959). *Mourning and melancholia.* In *Collected Papers,* vol. 4, 152–70. New York: Basic Books.

Garber, J., & Hollon, S. D. (1980). Universal versus personal helplessness in depression: Belief in uncontrollability or incompetence? *Journal of Abnormal Psychology,* 89, 56–66.

Hawkins, W. L.; French, L. C.; Crawford, B. D.; & Enzle, M. E. (1988). Depressed affect and time perspective. *Journal of Abnormal Psychology,* 97, 275–80.

Hiroto, D. S. (1974). Locus of control and learned helplessness. *Journal of Experimental Psychology,* 102, 187–93.

Hollon, S. D., & Kendall, P. C. (1980). Cognitive self-statements in depression: Development of an automatic thoughts questionnaire. *Cognitive therapy and Research,* 4, 383–95.

Jones, R. G. (1968). *A factored measure of Ellis' irrational belief system.* Wichita, Kans.: Test Systems.

Krantz, S. E. (1985). When depressive cognitions reflect negative realities. *Cognitive Therapy and Research,* 9, 595–610.

Lewinsohn, P. M.; Mischel, W.; Chaplin, W.; & Barton, R. (1980). Social competency and depression: The role of illusory self-perceptions. *Journal of Abnormal Psychology,* 89, 203–12.

Maier, S. F., & Seligman, M. E. P. (1976). Learned helplessness: Theory and evidence. *Journal of Experimental Psychology: General,* 105, 3–46.

Mayo, P. R. (1967). Some psychological changes associated with improvement in depression. *British Journal of Psychiatry,* 188, 671–73.

Meyersburg, H. A.; Ablon, S. L.; & Kotin, J. (1974). A reverberating psychic mechanism in the depressive processes. *Psychiatry,* 37, 372–86.

Nelson, R. E. (1977). Irrational beliefs in depression. *Journal of Consulting and Clinical Psychology,* 45, 1190–91.

Pacht, A. R. (1984). Reflections on perfection. *American Psychologist,* 39, 386–90.

Peterson, C., & Villanova, P. (1988). An expanded attributional style questionnaire. *Journal of Abnormal Psychology,* 97, 87–89.

Robbins, P. R., & Tanck, R. H. (1984). Sex differences in problems related to depression. *Sex Roles,* 11, 703–7.

Rotter, J. B. (1960). Generalized expectancies for internal versus external control of reinforcement. *Psychological Monographs,* 80, 609.

Smith, T. W., & Greenberg, J. (1981). Depression and self-focused attention. *Motivation and Emotion,* 5, 323–31.

Snyder, C. R. (1984, September). Excuses, excuses. *Psychology Today,* 18, 50–55.

Swallow, S. R., & Kuiper, N. A. (1988). Social comparison and negative self-evaluations: An application to depression. *Clinical Psychology Review,* 8, 55–76.

Wenzlaff, R. M., & Grozier, S. A. (1988). Depression and the magnification of failure. *Journal of Abnormal Psychology,* 97, 90–93.

Wortman, C. B., & Silver, R. C. (1989). The myths of coping with loss. *Journal of Consulting and Clinical Psychology,* 57, 349–57.

5. The Roots of Depression: A Look at Childhood Experiences

It is axiomatic that one's past experiences influence what one is today. The influence of childhood experiences seems particularly important, for that is where formative personality patterns are laid down. It seems reasonable to search for long-range causes of adult depression in child development and especially in the pattern of parent-child relationships.

Some patients enter therapy with this idea in mind; they assume that there are deep underlying causes for their depressed feelings and anticipate that the therapist will spend considerable time delving into their childhood recollections trying to unearth these causes. The thinking may be that when these causes are uncovered, the depressive symptoms will disappear. This can be a somewhat romanticized view of therapy, for there are usually pressing problems that confront patients in their daily lives and that demand attention in therapy, problems that are currently having an impact on the patient's well being. Nonetheless, these patients do have a point. Understanding one's past often puts the depressive problem into a much clearer perspective.

As an illustration of this, a young woman, Alexandra, entered therapy. She was experiencing considerable anxiety and depression, and had serious problems relating to self-confidence. A failure in her most recent job had plunged her self-esteem to a low level. Alexandra's therapist explored her past history. She learned that Alexandra had previous experiences of failure and when new opportunities presented themselves, she had an expectation of failure. Alexandra and her therapist traced the idea that she couldn't succeed back through her school years to her early relationships with her parents and to her Aunt

Josie, with whom she used to spend her summers in the country. Her mother—who had been widowed when her husband died in an automobile crash—was overprotective, not letting Alexandra play in the street with other children. She was careful to see that Alexandra "wouldn't get hurt." Her mother was always saying "Don't do this" and "Don't do that." For her part, Josie was usually critical of the things Alexandra did and left her with the feeling that she couldn't do anything right. When Alexandra tried to help Josie in the kitchen or with her garden, she was left with the feeling that she was a klutz. During the course of therapy, Alexandra began to understand that these early experiences had thwarted the building of self-confidence. She realized that her current depression had a long history underlying it and was better able to understand her problem.

Theories of child development often make the assumption, implicitly if not explicitly, that successful experiences in an earlier phase of human development will increase the chances of successful experiences in later phases of development. Think of making a structure out of building blocks; if the lower blocks are placed correctly, the growing structure will be well supported. If the supporting blocks are badly placed, the structure may crumble. If the child fails to adapt well in early phases of development, there is an increased likelihood of trouble down the line. Obviously, there are many things that can happen in later experiences to mitigate the effects of early problems; there is no inevitability that developmental difficulties will lead to depression or other psychological problems. Nonetheless, a bad start is just that and could leave the child with handicaps in the race of life that lies ahead.

When we observe emotional difficulties in children, we consider a variety of possible causes. Among the chief suspects are parent-child relationships, for these relationships are of prime importance in providing the skills and understanding the child needs to negotiate the world about her or him. When there are failures in these all-important relationships, one may anticipate a greater chance for future problems.

The Concept of Attachment

In discussing parent-child relationships, let's begin with the very early days, the first year of life. One of the fundamental processes that occurs at this time is *attachment*. Attachment has been defined by such theorists as John Bowlby as any type of behavior in which an individual maintains closeness (usually physical nearness) with another individual who is perceived as more capable of dealing with the world.[1] One can see immediately that for the infant, attachment is all important as the infant is helpless, totally dependent on others for survival. Attachment in the infant is more than being fed, cleaned or clothed; it includes the physical comfort of being held and cuddled and the sense of security that comes with this contact.

The importance of cuddly contact was underscored by Harry Harlow's ingenious experiments with infant chimps. In these experiments, Harlow used different types of mechanical "surrogate mothers." One of the mothers was soft and cloth covered, but provided no nursing; the other was simple wire mesh with a bottle. Given a choice, the infant chimps preferred the cloth mother without feeding to the wire mesh mother with feeding.

Observations by Rene Spitz, John Bowlby and others in England during and following the Second World War also point to the importance of attachment and the hazards of prolonged separation from the mother for the normal emotional development of the child. Children who experienced prolonged separation from their mothers went through a sequence of distress reactions. The infants began by protesting; they were angry. Later, they began to show despair. Finally, they became detached and did not seek the comfort of adults. The normal attachment bonds, which offer a secure base for dealing with the world, had been severely damaged.

The writings of Bowlby were very influential in stimulating interest in attachment. Researchers following in Bowlby's footsteps have delineated several phases in the process of attachment. In the beginning there is a *preattachment phase*, which lasts for the first eight to twelve weeks of life. By the age of two or three months, the infant begins groping for attachments, usually developing a preference for being close to the mother. Around the age of six months, a primary pattern of attachment is well established; the young child uses this relationship as a base from which to explore and test his or her environs. It is something like a safe port in uncharted seas. Eventually, as the child develops more understanding and capabilities, the child becomes less dependent.[2]

---

[1]*Bowlby (1982), p. 668.*
[2]*For a discussion of research relating to attachment, see the articles by Goldsmith & Alansky (1987) and by Cicchetti (1987).*

Mary Ainsworth, who has made singular contributions to the study of attachment, provides us with a descriptive analysis of this early attachment process.

> At birth, the infant is equipped with a repertoire of species-characteristic behaviors that promote proximity to a caregiver. Most conspicuous among these are signaling behaviors, such as crying, that operate to activate caregiving behavior, attracting the caregiver to come near. At first, these attachment behaviors are simply emitted, rather than being directed toward any specific person, but gradually the baby begins to discriminate one person from another and to direct attachment behavior differentially.
>
> At about the middle of the infant's first year, a new phase of development may be identified. A number of important changes occur more or less simultaneously. These include the emergence of locomotion and directed reaching and grasping, which enable proximity-keeping behavior to become more active, effective, and "goal-oriented." Furthermore, the baby forms his or her first inner representation of the principal caregiver, having attained some capacity for believing that the caregiver exists even when not present to perception, and with this achievement comes the onset of separation distress when the caregiver leaves the infant. At this point, the baby is capable of attachment and is very likely to have become attached not only to his or her mother figure, but to one or a few other familiar persons as well.[3]

The implications of attachment and separation for the child's emotional health are being systematically studied in the psychological laboratory using a procedure developed by Ainsworth and her colleagues, called the *strange situation*. The procedure consists of a number of episodes that last about three minutes each. In the beginning segments, the mother and her infant child go into an unfamiliar room. There, they are joined by a woman who is a stranger to them. The mother leaves the infant with the woman. After a few minutes the mother returns and the stranger leaves. Then the mother departs also, leaving the infant alone. While these sequences take place, the infant's reactions are monitored. Researchers note how the infant reacts both to the separation from the mother and to the reunion with her. The researchers note whether the infant seeks contact with the mother and the stranger, whether there is avoidance and whether the infant engages in searching behavior while separated. The observers evaluate the attachment relationship as to whether it is "secure" or "insecure" in various ways. For the great majority of children, the relationship is evaluated as secure.

[3]*Ainsworth (1989), p. 710.*

Attachment theorists believe that the way a mother behaves toward her child affects the security of the child's attachment. In observing the mother's behavior, they ask such questions as, How responsive is she to the child's crying? Does she spend time being close to the child? Does she hold the child when the child expresses this desire? Is she affectionate? Does she appear positive when she talks to the child? Using the child's behavior in the strange situation as a basis for measurement, researchers have found that as the theorists anticipated, the attachment relationships of infants of responsive, sensitive mothers tend to be more secure. While the mother's caretaking behavior is not the only factor that makes a difference in the security of the child, it is significant.

One may wonder what the long-range significance of the kind of behavior monitored in the strange situation is. Can one make predictions about what the child will be like a number of years later when she or he is well along in school? While the jury is still out on this question, at least one long-range study being carried out on children born into high-risk families (e.g., parents who are single mothers, disadvantaged economically) suggests that early attachment ratings are harbingers of future behavior. The attachment observations were made in the strange situation in 1975 and as of this date, the children who were evaluated as securely attached are more confident, enthusiastic and popular with their peers.[4] The suggestion is that a secure early attachment between mother and child promotes positive emotional development in the child.

Troublesome Patterns in Children

A current view in the child development literature articulated by Sidney Blatt is that two patterns of parent-child relations seem particularly related to the development of depressive tendencies. The first pattern follows from the research on attachment and separation. In this scenario, the child develops a fear of abandonment by the mother and of not being loved by her. Such fears may lead to exaggerated dependency on others for support and satisfaction in life, to feelings of helplessness and fears of being on one's own. Depression with these characteristics has been termed *anaclitic depression*.

---

[4]*See Adler (1989). The study cited is being carried out by Byron Egeland and his colleagues.*

Following through on this idea, we might deduce that if separation from parents in childhood increases vulnerability to later depression, the death of a parent would be linked to later depression in the child and perhaps in the adult as well. Researchers examining biographical information and depression inventory scores of adults have found an association between the death of a parent during the patient's childhood and current levels of depression.[5] The death of the father may have as much of an effect on subsequent depression as the death of the mother.

The second pattern of parent-child relationships that seems to foster depression is one in which the relationship is characterized by excessive negative parental control. In this pattern, parents are often hostile and deprecatory and inconsistent in offering affection. Under these conditions, the child learns to feel unworthy and unlovable and may develop a strong sense of guilt and a pattern of self-criticism. The child may feel she or he has not lived up to expectations and may develop a need for super-striving in order to prove her- or himself. Depression that emphasizes these problems has been called *introjective depression.*

When adult depressed patients are asked about their memories of the way their parents raised them, their reports often sound like the introjective pattern. In reviewing the studies on this topic, researchers Edward McCranie and Judith Bass wrote, "Considered together, these studies suggest that depression proneness in general is influenced by parental child-rearing practicies that combine elements of rejection, inconsistent expressions of affection, and strict control. Such parental behaviors could be expected to hinder the development of normal self-esteem in the child, resulting in an increased vulnerability to generalized feelings of helplessness and failure."[6]

As an example, in one study women who had experienced depression and women who had not were asked to agree or disagree with a number of statements describing their mothers. The women who had experienced depressive problems more often endorsed statements that portrayed their mothers as critical and demanding, such as, "Mother wanted me to be different," "Mother felt many things about my performance should be corrected," "I couldn't live up to Mother's expectations," "Mother honored my brothers' and sisters' requests more than mine."[7]

[5] *See Nelson (1982).*
[6] *See McCranie & Bass (1984), p. 7.*
[7] *Cofer & Winterborn (1980), p. 313. See in particular table 5.*

We must introduce a note of caution here because these studies use retrospective accounts, memories of what things were like in childhood. Like perception, memory is selective; we remember some things and not others. And there are many studies that show that depressed emotion can influence what one recalls. People who are depressed often show a bias toward recalling what is unpleasant. This bias poses an obvious problem in interpreting retrospective accounts.

There is yet another problem with retrospective studies, particularly concerning early childhood. Many people have difficulty remembering very much about this period. In conducting research on this problem, we have found that recall is often very poor. For the first three years of life, about half of our subjects couldn't remember *anything.* About one in ten subjects couldn't recall anything through age six. To appreciate the difficulties that might be involved in retrospective accounts, think back to your very early memories. What do you recall?

Going beyond these two patterns, we know that parents who are angry, or worse, cruel and abusive, can leave emotional scars on children. The effects of physical abuse of children are found in poor performance in school, conduct problems, anxiety and social withdrawal, as well as depressed reactions.

In discussing their study of children who were inpatients in a psychiatric facility, Alan Kazdin and his colleagues reported that children who had been physically abused "evince higher levels of depression and hopelessness and lower self-esteem than do nonabused patients . . . and viewed themselves and their futures more negatively than did children without phsyical abuse."[8]

Another source of potential problems are homes in which there is a high level of parental discord. Such homes are a fertile environment for children to germinate the seeds of emotional difficulties. It can be a severe strain on children to witness a declared or undeclared war between their parents. Children who go through the divorce of their parents not only experience this tension, but they experience the subsequent loss of separation. It is no wonder that anger, depressed reactions and withdrawal are among the common reactions observed in children to the divorce of their parents.[9] There are parallels here with the reactions

[8]*Kazdin et al. (1985), p. 304.*
[9]*For a discussion of the psychological effects of divorce on children, see Hetherington (1989).*

described by Bowlby when attachments were severed in very young children.

The Importance of Confidence-Building Activities

One of the important aspects of early attachment relationships is that they give the child a secure base with which to explore his or her world and begin to develop competence in mastering the environment. This builds feelings of confidence. Competence and confidence are very important in becoming a fully effective individual. The home atmosphere that promotes these tendencies will help the child develop a sense of self-esteem. The home atmosphere that does not may promote learned helplessness, which increases the risk of a depressive reaction.

To grow in competence and gain the confidence that comes with it, children need the opportunity to explore, to try and to succeed. Parents like Alexandra's mother and Aunt Josie, whose repetitive messages to the child are "no," "don't," and "you can't," are not providing her this opportunity. The parent who is impatient with the child, who takes over and says, "Here, I'll do it," when the task is within the child's capabilities, prevents the child from developing a sense of mastery in dealing with her or his environment.

Confidence-building activities are vital in the formative years. In addition to the early home environment, the school is an important setting for this kind of learning. Some children prosper in school, but not all do. Think back to your classrooms in elementary and junior high school. Do you remember some of the very bright kids in the class? It seems like their hands were always flying high to answer the teacher's questions and the teacher called on them time and again. The children were praised— their marks were glowing. Whatever else was happening in their lives, these children knew they were good students. But what about the children who were not as quick? Who praised them? Chances are many such students faded into the woodwork and were ignored. And what about the children who really had to struggle in school? Some of these children took a psychological beating.

The message of years of being ignored or worse, put down, is cumulative and clear: "You're not competent—you don't measure up." If the child has compensating talents like athletic ability or artistic or mechanical skills, these can go a long way as a self-confidence booster.

The important thing is that children need to experience success as they grow up.

Self-confidence comes not only from academic success but from interpersonal success as well. Children who do not develop social skills tend to experience rejection and loneliness. Poorly developed social skills in children can be a harbinger of possible future psychological and social difficulties. Researchers have found that children who experience a "double whammy," having both poorer academic and social skills, are more likely to be depressed.[10]

We are sketching a picture of what is often a subclinical depression in children. Picture a child who is neglected or rejected by his peers and not doing well academically. Such a child is unlikely to feel very good about himself. Teachers can often spot such a lonely, unhappy child. The child's classmates may be even better at it. The consensual opinion of children about their classmates is often revealing.

It is possible to obtain such opinions in research. To cite an example, using a "peer nomination" technique, Monroe Lefkowitz and Edward Tesiny gathered groups of children into a schoolroom and read aloud a series of descriptive statements that included such items as, "Who often plays alone?" "Who thinks they are bad?" "Who says they can't do things?" "Who doesn't have much fun?" "Who thinks others don't like them?" "Who often looks lonely?"[11] The children's tasks were to think about their classmates and check all the names on their class roster that best fit the description.

What happened in Lefkowitz's and Tesiny's study was that most of the children in the class received *no votes* at all. Most of the children were not viewed by their peers as depressed. However, there were some children who were clearly picked out by their peers as depressed.

When the researchers compared these "nominated" children with their classmates, they uncovered some interesting findings. First, the nominated children were rated by themselves as depressed. They recognized that they had a problem. These children also had lower self-esteem on psychological testing. Like adults who are depressed, they more often saw the sources of gratification in life as under external control. They were more often absent from school and performed less well on reading and math achievement tests.

[10]*See, for example, Coleg (1990).*
[11]*Lefkowitz & Tesiny (1980), p. 44.*

The psychology of these children—their lowered self-esteem and external view of control of gratification seems very similar to the patterns we saw earlier in depressed adults. Do depressed children also show some of the other thinking patterns typical of depressed adults, such as overgeneralization and a tendency to blame oneself?

Harold Leitenberg and his colleagues carried out an interesting study, which addressed this question. They presented hypothetical situations to children concerning three areas of their lives—social, academic and athletic. Following the hypothetical situations, they offered a negative thought pattern type of reaction. For example: "You call one of the kids in your class to talk about your math homework. He/she says, 'I can't talk to you now, my father needs to use the phone.' You think, 'He/she didn't want to talk to me.'" And, "Your cousin calls you to ask if you would like to go on a long bike ride. You think, 'I probably won't be able to keep up and people will make fun of me.'" The children were asked to respond to each situation using a scale ranging from "not at all like I would think" to "almost exactly like I would think."[12] The results were revealing. Similar to findings of the peer nomination study, the researchers found that most of the children did not believe that they would usually react to these situations with such negative interpretations. Negative thought patterns were not typical for young children.

The researchers reported some interesting observations. First, when negative thought patterns arose, they were most likely to arise in the social area. Young children were more likely to overgeneralize or catastrophize from incidents in their peer relationships than from events in the classroom or athletic field. Second, very young children were more prone to catastrophize and personalize mishappenings than older children. As the researchers suggest, very young children lack the experience to understand that mistakes and failures do not necessarily have dire consequences. Young children may blow the situation out of proportion. Third, and most important for our inquiry, the children who showed tendencies to overgeneralize, catastrophize and hold themselves responsible for bad outcomes were more likely to report depressed feelings. This is the same pattern we see in adults.

These findings for children then are in some respects a mirror for what we observe in adults. Most children do not have negative thinking patterns; those who do are more likely to be depressed. Most adults do

[12]*Leitenberg et al. (1986), pp. 529–30.*

not think that way either. Those who do are more likely to feel depressed. These parallel findings recall the idea of building blocks—the impact of one stage of development on the next. The child is indeed the father of the man. The elements of adult depression are forming in the child. One sees loneliness, low self-esteem, perception of external control, a tendency to overgeneralize and catastrophize failures and blame oneself. All of these adult tendencies may be observed in vulnerable children, presumably resulting from the interplay of genetics and psychologically punishing environments. When environmental stressors become too difficult to handle, a depressive reaction may develop—even in children.

In carrying out research on the way children evaluate good and bad events, Martin Seligman and his colleagues arrived at a similar conclusion. They wrote, "children with depressive symptoms share some characteristics of adults with depressive symptoms. Both have an attributional style in which bad events are seen as caused by internal, stable, and global factors. Both may be put at risk for future depression by processing information about bad events through this insidious attributional style."[13]

The potential for depression that is developed in childhood is carried into adolescence. Biological changes that take place at puberty create profound changes in the child's life. Rapid physical and sexual maturation accompanied by increased independence from parents generate considerable uncertainty and stress. Psychological vulnerabilities that may have been created in childhood can lead to poorer skills for coping with these stresses, making adjustment more difficult. Many adolescents experience periods of mild to moderate depression.

Difficulties in relationships within one's own family are often the biggest problem for adolescents and sometimes are related to depressive episodes. Tensions in the relationship of the adolescent and parents can create problems for both parties. Problems in social relationships are another prime source of emotional downers for teenagers as acceptance by one's peer group assumes a very high place in the world of adolescence. The depressed symptoms of the adolescent are in most respects similar to those of adults. In addition to the litany of depressed symptoms we have outlined earlier, the depressed teenager is likely to have trouble with school work and get poorer grades.

Researchers studying teenagers with depressive symptoms have

[13]*Seligman et al. (1984), p. 238.*

reported that there are some differences in the way boys and girls show their depressed feelings. Adolescent boys who are depressed are more likely than girls to appear antagonistic, unrestrained and discontented. They feel worried and alienated. They often get into trouble in school and don't do well in their school work. Depressed adolescent girls also feel alienated and angry, but these feelings usually are less observable in the girls' behavior. Depressed adolescent girls may appear passive. They may become introspective and frequently have problems with self-esteem.[14]

While problems within the family circle and difficulties relating to peers are often sources of stress in adolescence, it is important to recognize that both family and peers may also act as a buffer against stress for the teenager. The teenager who feels he or she is part of a together-functioning family where people feel connected and care about each other has a real advantage in coping with the problems of adolescence. Having good friends is also a very important source of support for the teenager.

There are a number of growth experiences — "developmental tasks" we think of as important in adolescence — competencies that we normally expect teenagers to develop during this important phase of life. We think of such things as gaining a substantial measure of independence from one's parents, finishing high school and beginning to date. Successful experiences in adolescence promote successful experiences in adulthood to follow. Failure to develop these skills may not only be associated with a troublesome adolescence but could lay the groundwork for future difficulties.

BIBLIOGRAPHY

Adler, T. (1989, April). Infant is father to the child, studies show. *American Psychological Association Monitor*, 7.

Ainsworth, M. D. S. (1989). Attachments beyond infancy. *American Psychologist*, 44, 709–16.

Barnes, G. E., & Prosen, H. (1985). Parental death and depression. *Journal of Abnormal Psychology*, 94, 64–69.

Blatt, S. J. (1974). Levels of object representation in anaclitic and introjective depression. *Psychoanalytic Study of the Child*, 29, 107–57.

[14]*See Gjerde et al. (1988). Gender differences are discussed on pp. 482–83.*

Blechman, E. A.; McEnroe, M. J.; Carella, E. T.; & Audette, D. P. (1986). Childhood competence and depression. *Journal of Abnormal Psychology*, 95, 223–27.

Bowlby, J. (1982). Attachment and loss: Retrospect and prospect. *American Journal of Orthopsychiatry*, 52, 664–78.

Burbach, D. J., & Borduin, C. M. (1986). Parent-child relations and the etiology of depression: A review of methods and findings. *Clinical Psychology Review*, 6, 133–53.

Cicchetti, D. (1987). Developmental psychopathology in infancy: Illustration from the study of maltreated youngsters. *Journal of Consulting and Clinical Psychology*, 55, 837–45.

Cofer, D. H., & Winterborn, J. R. (1980). Personality characteristics of formerly depressed women. *Journal of Abnormal Psychology*, 89, 309–14.

Coleg, E. A. (1990). Relation of social and academic competence to depressive symptoms in childhood. *Journal of Abnormal Psychology*, 99, 422–29.

Fisher-Beckfield, D., & McFall, R. M. (1982). Development of a competence inventory for college men and evaluation of relationships between competence and depression. *Journal of Consulting and Clinical Psychology*, 50, 699–705.

Gjerde, P. F.; Block, J.; & Block, J. (1988). Depressive symptoms and personality during late adolescence: Gender differences in externalization–internalization of symptom expression. *Journal of Abnormal Psychology*, 97, 475–86.

Goldsmith, H. H., & Alansky, J. A. (1987). Maternal and infant temperamental predictors of attachment: A meta-analytic review. *Journal of Consulting and Clinical Psychology*, 55, 805–16.

Harlow, H. F. (1958). The nature of love. *American Psychologist*, 13, 673–85.

Hetherington, E. M.; Hagan, M. S.; & Anderson, E. T. (1989). Marital transitions: A child's perspective. *American Psychologist*, 44, 303–12.

Kazdin, A. E.; Moser, J.; Colbus, D.; & Bell, R. (1985). Depressive symptoms among physically abused and psychiatrically disturbed children. *Journal of Abnormal Psychology*, 94, 298–307.

Lefkowitz, M. M., & Tesiny, E. P. (1980). Assessment of childhood depression. *Journal of Consulting and Clinical Psychology*, 48, 43–50.

Leitenberg, H.; Yost, L. W.; & Carroll-Wilson, M. (1986). Negative cognitive errors in children: Questionnaire development, normative data, and comparisons between children with and without self-reported symptoms of depression, low self-esteem, and evaluation anxiety. *Journal of Consulting and Clinical Psychology*, 54, 528–36.

McCranie, E. W., & Bass, J. D. (1984). Childhood family antecedents of dependency and self-criticism: Implications for depression. *Journal of Abnormal Psychology*, 93, 3–8.

Nelson, G. (1982). Parental death during childhood and adult depression: Some additional data. *Social Psychiatry*, 17, 37–42.

Reynolds, W. M., & Coats, K. I. (1982). Depression in adolescents: Incidence, depth, and correlates. Paper presented at 10th International Congress, International Association of Child and Adolescent Psychiatry and Allied Professions, Dublin, Ireland.

Robbins, P. R., & Tanck, R. (1987). *Personal growth: A teenager's guide.* Portland, Maine: J. Weston Walch.

Seligman, M. E. P.; Peterson, C.; Kaslow, N. J.; Tanenbaum, R. L.; Alloy, L. B.; & Abramson, L. Y. (1984). Attributional style and depressive symptoms among children. *Journal of Abnormal Psychology,* 93, 235–38.

Spitz, R. A. (1946). Anaclitic depression. *Psychoanalytic Study of the Child,* 2, 313–42.

Walker, L. S., & Greene, J. W. (1987). Negative life events, psychosocial resources, and psychophysiological symptoms in adolescents. *Journal of Clinical Child Psychology,* 16, 29–36.

6. Stress and Depressed Mood

It is very common for depressed moods to develop during periods of stress. Though not always the case, when depressed people are questioned about what was going on in their lives when they began to feel depressed, they often relate stories of being under stress. Both clinical observation and research evidence point to the conclusion that when people have a vulnerability toward depression, stressful events in life may trigger a depressed reaction.[1]

In describing their model of the depressive process, H. A. Meyersburg and his colleagues present some case material that illustrates the way mounting stress can precipitate a depressive reaction. Consider Judith, a 40-year-old woman who once had a depressive episode during college but had been relatively free of problems since that time. One day her husband informed her that "he had a girlfriend and filed for a divorce. When the decree was finalized, Judith moved away with her three children. She felt overwhelmed, extremely anxious, and unable to care for herself or them."[2] She was subsequently hospitalized for depression. "In discussions with other patients and staff, Judith spoke about a vague, diffuse anxiety, helplessness and neediness."[3]

Or take the case of Sally, a woman in her early twenties. Sally came from a family in which both parents had depressive problems, suggesting that Sally was at increased risk. The precipitating stressor in Sally's case was a romantic relationship. Sally became involved with a young man

---

[1]*There are many studies that indicate that stress can be a precipitating factor in depression. The studies of Benjaminsen (1981) and of Lloyd (1980) are examples.*
[2]*Meyersburg et al. (1974), p. 384.*
[3]*Meyersburg et al. (1974), p. 384.*

whom she found attractive, but at the same time she was frightened of sexual experience. As the relationship developed, her anxiety mounted. She rebuffed him and he broke off their relationship. Following the breakup, she became severely depressed.

Meyersburg and his colleagues view stress as having an overwhelming effect on a vulnerable person, precipitating depression. Indeed, a very stressful event can have a depressive effect on many people who are normally resilient. A traumatic experience such as rape will often leave in its wake a depressive reaction that may persist for months.[4] The emotional effects of combat may linger for years.

When we talk about stress, we often think about anxiety. Anxious and depressed feelings are not identical, but they are highly related. We usually think of anxiety as being worried or feeling tense. Often, anxiety has an anticipatory, foreboding quality. It is a feeling that comes with thinking about upcoming events that may be unpleasant or uncertain. Anxiety is that jittery feeling before taking an exam, giving a speech or calling up someone new for a date.

Like the feeling of depression, the feelings of anxiety are uncomfortable. The sympathetic nervous system is active. During acute anxiety, one sweats, the heart races and breathing becomes more difficult. Periods of anxiety are often accompanied by the same kind of physical complaints that are associated with depression—headaches, dizziness, nausea, and diarrhea. These two types of uncomfortable emotions—feeling anxious and depressed—may follow each other in tandem, like sequential musical notes, but often occur together. A person who experiences one emotion is likely to report the other.[5]

In studies of clinical populations, one often finds the two types of problems coexisting. Patients who are diagnosed as having an anxiety disorder often have depressive problems, while patients diagnosed as depressed often have significant anxiety problems. To cite an example, James Leckman and his colleagues studied a sample of 133 patients who had been diagnosed as depressed and found that 77 of the patients also

---

[4]*See Frank et al. (1979).*

[5]*Aaron Beck and his colleagues have been conducting research that attempts to clarify the differences between anxiety and depression. In one study, for example, David Clark, Beck and Bonnie Stewart reported, "The depressed patients reported significantly more hopelessness, lower self-worth, and more negative thoughts involving loss and past failure. The anxious group, on the other hand, had significantly more thoughts of anticipated harm and danger." Clark, et al. (1990).*

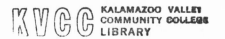

had problems relating to anxiety such as panic disorder, generalized anxiety disorder or agoraphobia.

We all feel anxious at times and most of us go through periods when we experience stress. Many people are able to handle stress relatively well. Some people even welcome it. Are you the sort of person that would enjoy free-fall parachuting from airplanes or scaling high mountains? Many people, however, have problems dealing with stress. For some people, when stress mounts and becomes difficult to handle, depression may set in.

It is my belief that when stress becomes uncomfortable and *no solution is in sight to change things,* depression is most likely to occur. When depression persists and becomes a lingering event, there may be some changes in focus—from the external stressors more onto the self. The focus may change from "The situation is awful" to "The situation is awful and *I can't function.*" A kind of psychological paralysis sets in. One of the effects of this immobilization is that the person may tend to avoid the stress situation. He may take sick leave from work, drop that difficult course in school or avoid social contacts. Depression in this sense functions like a psychological defense, protecting the ego from further stress. The price exacted is pain and suffering of another kind.

Depressed People and Stress

Everyday observation tells us that some people can tolerate a great deal of stress without becoming depressed while other people cannot. Why is this so? What accounts for this difference?

The findings from research suggest that there is no single answer to this question. The answers probably lie in biological differences—some people have a genetic makeup that makes them more vulnerable to depression, in childhood experience, in psychological differences in the way people evaluate stress-arousing situations and in the way they cope with these situations. We have previously considered the role of genetic differences and childhood experiences. Let us now examine the way people evaluate stress-provoking situations and the ways in which they respond to them.

Two people can size up a situation that is a problem and view it quite differently. Consider a problem that might happen on the job—there's some unfinished work sitting on the desk. Dave might think it's extremely important to get it done. He may think, "If I don't work late tonight and finish it—no matter how long it takes—the boss and my co-workers will think I'm not up to the job." In contrast, Bill might think, "The work will still be there tomorrow. The world won't come to an end if it takes an extra day. If I wait until tomorrow, I'm not going to lose my job and the company isn't going to go broke."

The company may be much happier with Dave's attitude than Bill's, but if that is Dave's *characteristic approach to life*, he may be setting himself up for trouble. He may be overevaluating or inflating the importance of what he is doing—not distinguishing between what is important and what is not, where a maximum effort is really needed. He may also be investing too much of his self-esteem in the activity. If things don't work out, he'll take the setback harder.

Research has suggested that people who become depressed tend to inflate the importance of the problems they face, feeling there is more at stake and more to lose. Their self-esteem is more often on the line.[6] When higher stakes are placed on an outcome, insecurity and anxiety are likely to develop during the process of resolving the problem. The person is more likely to experience the symptoms of stress—edginess, irritability and physical complaints.

If the situation is confrontational, involving another person, there is a higher chance of the stressed individual reacting emotionally. As the confrontation mounts, anger mounts. He or she may explode in an emotional outburst or the anger may be vented later at someone else who just happens to be around. If the problem is not resolved in a satisfactory way—and that happens to almost everyone—more hurt and disappointment may be experienced. High stakes can lead to a greater sense of loss and lowered self-esteem. Depressed people often report that their feelings are easily hurt, that they take things hard. Part of the reason for this reaction is that they have mentally turned hills into mountains. When the hill collapses, it seems like the mountain has collapsed.

When responding to stress, persons who become depressed are less likely to cope with the situation by taking the kind of rational, concerted action needed to solve the problems. Instead of engaging in problem-solving behavior, they often become bogged down in inaction and self-analysis. Wishful thinking and avoidance sometimes provide a defense for the faltering ego, but obviously have only limited value for the long

[6]*See Folkman & Lazarus (1986), p. 110, table 2.*

term.[7] If the depressed reaction, itself, becomes disabling, it may act as a defense against having to deal with the stressors beleaguering the person. When one is disabled, one is not expected to deal with problems. Such a defense, of course, only extends one's misery.

Researchers have accumulated a large amount of data that suggests that major changes in life act as stressors and may trigger depression in those who are vulnerable. By major life changes, we mean such events as developing a serious illness, changing jobs, moving to a different part of the country, getting divorced, having a child or losing a close friend. Researchers have compiled lists of such events, put them in the form of a questionnaire and found that people who have been going through major life changes are more vulnerable to emotional problems including depression. In one study, depressed men and women reported twice as many of these events as subjects in a control group.[8]

One of the key elements in many of these changes is loss. When a young man or woman goes away to college, for example, it is a challenging experience with great potential for personal growth, but it also means separation from long-standing sources of security — from parents, friends and neighborhood. Separation and loss can be very painful.

Ellen's experience is a good illustration of this. Ellen was a student in one of our research projects who found the transition to a large urban university very difficult and reported she was experiencing very high stress. She had previously boarded at a small all girls' school where she had lots of friends and close-knit relationships. The small classes had allowed an opportunity for students to discuss issues with their instructors and Ellen had found the atmosphere academically stimulating. Now her classes were held in large lecture halls, sometimes with hundreds of students. She disliked this change and missed her old friends badly.

Breakups in romantic relationships are one of the most painful of human experiences. It is the stuff that novels are made of, the basis of folk ballads and popular songs. Breaking up is also a source of countless

---

[7]*There have been a number of studies that relate techniques people use to cope with stress to feelings of depression. An example would be the studies carried out by Charles Holahan and Rudolf Moos. They assessed their subjects on a number of measures including coping techniques, then followed the subjects for several years. They reported, "We have found that personality characteristics that involve more self-confidence and more easygoing disposition, more family support, and fewer avoidant coping strategies predict lower levels of depression." Holahan & Moos (1991).*

[8]*See Billings et al. (1983), pp. 125–26.*

depressive reactions. Research has demonstrated that having a network of strong, supportive relationships seems to act as a barrier against depression. The loss of such ties is difficult to cope with.[9]

The observation that the experience of loss is often implicated in depression is, of course, not a new idea. As we indicated, Freud recognized the importance of loss in triggering depression many years ago in his essay *Mourning and Melancholia*. The theme has been amplified by Bowlby and others. However, it should be pointed out that there is no inevitability that loss—or other types of stressors will bring on a depressive reaction. Many people who experience the loss of a spouse or paralyzing injuries show little evidence of depressed reactions after the event or experience noticeable depressive problems later on.[10] It is not only the big changes in life that increase one's risk of experiencing a depressive reaction; it is also the seemingly unremitting pounding away of everyday problems. Roland Tanck and I asked college students to look over a checklist of problems that students might typically encounter (e.g., not doing well at school, having conflicts with parents, being short of money) and to check the problems that they were currently experiencing. We found that the more problems the students checked, the higher they scored on the measure of depression. One problem might not get you down, but three, or four or five? In a somewhat similar vein, A. D. Kanner and his colleagues developed a questionnaire that measures daily hassles, events like experiencing traffic noise, preparing meals and having to wait. The more hassles people reported, the greater the chance they felt depressed.

These studies point to the role of the everyday stressors in our lives in triggering depression. And where better to look for such stressors than in our places of work, at school, in our marriages and families, and our relationships. These, our primary sources of joy and fulfillment in life, can also be causes of stress, playing a part in the development of depressed reactions.

[9]*For a review of research on the buffering effects of social support see Cohen and Wills (1985).*

[10]*While the evidence indicates that many people are able to cope with serious losses without experiencing depression, the chances of becoming depressed nonetheless are increased. A study by Patrick Shrout and his colleagues (1989) suggests that experiencing fateful losses such as the death of a spouse or child, the loss of a home or job or being unable to find treatment for a serious illness raises the odds of becoming depressed. A study by Stanley Murrell and Samuel Himmelfarb (1989) indicates that the depressive effects of bereavement in older adults tend to dissipate within a year.*

Stress on the Job

In the early years of the twentieth century, it was not uncommon for people to work 12- or 14-hour days, six days a week. For many people, one's work and one's life were almost synonymous. Now that people typically work 40 hours a week or less on a job (we are excluding workaholics), the job has become more a part of life rather than its near totality. Still the workplace is very important. Jobs provide much of what we find meaningful and satisfying in life, both in terms of daily activities and human relationships. Along with these benefits, a person's job can be a source of stress.

If you think about your own job experiences, you could probably develop your own list of stress-provoking situations that relate to work. There are probably not too many jobs that are completely devoid of stress. And some jobs are inherently stressful, posing real elements of physical danger. A police officer walking the beat in a crime-ridden neighborhood and a fire fighter trying to put out the flames in a collapsing building are obvious examples.

Stress may come from many sources in the workplace. Stress may arise from having responsibility for others. Consider an airline pilot with the lives of hundreds of people depending on her or his judgment or a surgeon performing an operation. Stress may be generated by the constraints of time when a job must be performed quickly. Picture an air traffic controller or a long distance telephone operator with a backup of calls. Stress may be generated by monotonous repetition. Think of an assembly line for automobiles or electronic products. Think of doing the same limited tasks, hour after hour after hour, day after day. Stress may be generated by noise. Imagine working near a pneumatic drill grinding into concrete or woking in a day care center full of noisy children. And stress may be generated by people. Have you ever had a boss that made life difficult for you? Have you ever worked with a person who you would just as soon took a one-way trip to Outer Mongolia?

There may be other sources of stress in a job. Consider low pay, little job security, lack of benefits, unfairness in promotion, sexual harassment, or how about a hassle just to get there, driving through rush hour traffic or commuting from miles away. And the job itself may conflict with other responsibilities such as running a home and taking care of the children.

There are various indicators that one might employ to "measure"

stress on the job: turnover rate, absenteeism, stress-related physical illness, depressed reactions and even suicide. Did you know that physicians, even psychiatrists, are hardly immune from these problems?
Women physicians have a considerably higher rate of suicide than other
adult women.[11] Who supports the people that support us in times of
trouble?

The stress experienced in the workplace may not only trigger depressed reactions in the worker but can impact the family. In a study of
job stress experienced by male blue collar workers, it was reported that
one-third of the men said their jobs had a negative effect on their
families. The sons of fathers who were experiencing job stress often had
poor relationships with their fathers and felt rejected and depressed.[12]

The financial cost of job-related stress is staggering. The cost of job
stress to industry is billions of dollars each year. As business pays about
half of the health care bills in this country, it makes economic sense for
business to do something about the stresses of the workplace, and this
is happening more and more. Among the programs that have been intro-
duced to help employees better cope with these stresses are mental
health counseling, provision of exercise facilities and the institution of
flex-time and day care centers to help employees better manage job and
nonjob responsibilities.

A term that has much in common with job-related depression is *burnout*. Have you ever felt this way or talked to someone complaining of
burnout? Typically, we think of a person who experiences burnout as
someone who has been on the job for a long time—often many years—has
done the same thing time after time, has lost interest and enthusiasm for
the work, feels drained and has little left to give. The images of work have
become negative and distasteful; the feelings include disillusionment and
anger, as well as the desire to avoid work.

Burnout from work is a kind of circumscribed depression: the source
of the problem is well defined. The depressed mood emanating from
work, however, can spill over to other areas of life and become a more
generalized malaise. Taking time off from work is an obvious antidote,
but it should be recognized that unless some changes are made in what
one is doing, either in one's job or in other areas of life to compensate
for the dissatisfactions of work, the person is likely to end up in the same

[11]*For a discussion of the emotional problems experienced by physicians, see Vaillant
et al. (1972).*
[12]*See Meer (1985).*

unpleasant situation. Career counseling may be helpful during the time-out period to discuss possible changes and new directions.

Having enumerated some of the unpleasant possibilities of stress on the job, we should say that there is something that is usually worse, and that is having no job at all. To be unemployed when you need to work or want to work can be demoralizing. People who leave a satisfying job without taking steps to find a better one may simply be jumping from the frying pan into the fire.

Unemployment is a situation in contemporary life that involves losses of all kinds: economic losses that force a reduction in the standard of living and restrict one's activities, loss of structure in one's daily life and often loss of self-esteem. During the Great Depression of the 1930s, a number of studies were carried out looking at the effects of unemployment. Researchers reported such psychological effects as the development of apathy, resignation, self-doubt, depression, lowered self-esteem and fatalistic beliefs.[13] The chances of such destructive psychological reactions happening probably increase as one experiences repeated failures with job applications.

The Marital Relationship

For many people, the marital relationship is an all-important source of companionship, support and stability. People who are married are likely to live longer and be happier than people who are not married. However, for many people, the marital relationship can be a source of stress, and this is very often the case in the lives of depressed people. Think for a moment about some of the bad marriages you have witnessed and you may have a picture in your mind of the type of marriage in which many depressed people find themselves. Researchers have examined the marital relationships of depressed people, comparing them with people who are not depressed and the findings are revealing. In the marriages of depressed people, there is more open conflict and hostility, and less expression of positive regard. There is also less problem-solving behavior. In commenting about these studies, James Coyne observes, "they [the studies] are remarkably consistent in indicating that these interactions are characterized by negative affect and tension."[14] In many instances,

---

[13]*See Feather & Barber (1983).*
[14]*Coyne (1985), p. 231.*

the spouses seem more like parties at war than partners for mutual benefit.

Depressed people often perceive the communications of their spouses as being negative. Part of this evaluation reflects the negative mind-set that depressed people have in evaluating the world about them. However, researchers who have directly observed depressed people interacting with their spouses report that much of this negativity in marital relationships is real.[15] The parties do not treat each other with regard.

In trying to understand the sources of this all too frequent smouldering environment, it is helpful to look at the situation from the perspective of both parties. For their part, depressed people feel lousy, not capable of doing the things that are usually expected of them. Yet they still may feel pressure to do these things—to work and to carry out their normal responsibilities. Depressed people may feel they are being pushed beyond what they can do, and this creates resentment.

Depression is an emotional illness, yet like most mental or emotional problems, it is less likely to arouse sympathy than a physical illness. Some people still respond to depression as if it were a weakness in character. The spouse may react with words like "You can stop it if you really want to." The depressed person may feel misunderstood and misjudged.

While depressed people often are burdened with guilt and self-recrimination, they are not above looking for other scapegoats for their problems. The depressed person can turn to the spouse and think "It's her fault," "he's not affectionate," "she doesn't care," or, "he's too angry," "she never listens," "we don't go any place." The list of marital complaints may be long and dreary. While these complaints often reflect reality, to some extent they may be brought on by the depressed person's own behavior.

Looking at the situation from the point of view of the other party in the marriage, it should be recognized that it is not an easy task to live with a person who is chronically depressed. In their conversations, depressed people are often pessimistic, run themselves down and present themselves as helpless and vulnerable. Studies have shown that even small doses of such behavior will turn off other people.[16] Many people do not find such behavior attractive and would rather avoid it. Daily

---

[15]*For example, Kowalik & Gotlib (1987).*
[16]*See, for example, Coyne (1976).*

doses of depressed behavior in the home are likely to arouse a wide range of emotions: compassion, concern, anxiety, feelings of being trapped, resentment and anger. At one time or another the spouses and families of depressed people may feel all of these emotions and it is not uncommon for the spouses of depressed persons to develop emotional problems of their own.[17]

Stress in Relationships

Difficult relationships with members of one's family, friends, neighbors or people at work can all be sources of stress. As a therapist, I hear such statements as, "I can't get along with my father — he's driving me crazy," or "I hate to go to my mother-in-law's house. We just don't get along." Such difficult relationships can add measurably to one's discomfort index. A troubled romantic relationship, however, may be in a class by itself for its potential to depress one's mood.

The plot of many Hollywood films during the heyday of the motion picture industry in the 1930s and 1940s was summed up in the formula, "boy meets girl, boy loses girl, boy gets girl." The plot of many real life romances is a little different. It is something like this: "boy meets girl, boy and girl become involved romantically and sexually, boy and girl break up, with one party — and sometimes both — bruised emotionally." Involvement and intimacy create strong feelings, which in this scenario are followed by feelings of loss. There was someone special in your life and that someone is gone.

It is often very hard for people to give up on busted romances. One can become "addicted" to the charms of another person in a manner that mimics addiction to drugs. Physical characteristics, voice, personality, sexual contact — the things that draw one to another person can exert a powerful hold and the desire may be very strong to hold on to an unworkable situation or to bring back what has gone. Memory may be selective, making the relationship seem better than it actually was. A little encouragement from the other party may revive hopes, not once but repeatedly, until it finally becomes clear that the pursuit is hopeless. The recognition that all is over often produces a depressed reaction. When a relationship is broken up, a person often feels broken up.

[17]*See Coyne et al. (1987).*

There are moving novels written about relationships that fail and about unrequited love. For example, *Of Human Bondage,* by W. Somerset Maugham, is a poignant novel depicting a hopeless attachment. In the therapist's office, one sees the grief and sadness that such romantic disappointment can bring. Time is usually a healer and one cautions against an inclination to give up on romance altogether, resolving not to risk being involved again and possibly hurt once more. To have a stable, supportive, gratifying relationship is much too important for men and women not to try again, to pick up the pieces and look for another person who seems right. Loneliness is a poor alternative.

Stress and the College Student

Our focus here is on college students, but much of what I have to say is applicable to the earlier years of school as well. Many students experience considerable stress during their years of primary and secondary school. When young men and women go to college, they often find themselves on their own for the first time, in a new and very different environment. While this experience is usually exciting, the students must cope with a variety of problems—issues relating to self-identity, career choice, reshaping their relationships with their parents and making new friends. These challenges may engender considerable discomfort, compounding the stress inherent in the way college as an institution is set up. College is like a road map. You must get from point A (admission) to point Z (graduation). The route involves showing mastery in many academic courses by passing exams and writing papers. These exams and papers for many students are *stress points* with anxiety often reaching peaks before and during exams.

This route has been traveled by millions, but many alumni would be surprised at the degree of stress existing today and the impact that it can have on the student's feeling of well being. Betty, a young woman, was studying sociology and anthropology at a metropolitan university. Betty came from a rural area where she, her widowed mother and three younger brothers formed a close-knit family. Betty had adjustment problems when she found herself alone in a very different kind of environment. She also had severe anxiety about how well she was performing in her classes. She worried constantly about term papers and exams, and obsessed about deadlines that were coming up. She would daydream that all her work was finished and she was back home with her family, or just brood about all the work that lay ahead of her. These thoughts became overwhelming and aggravated her ability to get started on anything. Physically, she did not feel well with frequent complaints of headaches, nausea, weakness and dizziness. She began to question whether the life-style she had fallen into made any sense and decided to talk with her psychology professor about the possibility of beginning therapy.

Mark was a career-oriented young man, who had his heart set on attending law school, preferably one of the prestigious law schools in the Northeast. In spite of his strong motivation, Mark was doing poorly as an undergraduate student and began to fear that he might not make the grades necessary to be admitted to the school of his choice. He thought what it would be like to fail his classes and started feeling depressed. When his exams were looming closer, he had dreams of being late for the exams. During the exams, he was very uptight and worried afterwards about his performance. He developed various physical complaints and had bouts of insomnia. He became irritable, had numerous arguments with his friends and family, and freely admitted that he was bothered by school and examinations.

Betty and Mark were students who participated in the studies Roland Tanck and I carried out using our diary technique. The diary included a question that asked, "Did you feel under any pressure or strain today relating to your schoolwork?" During the ten-day period covered by the diary, 95 percent of the students reported that they experienced at least one day of feeling such pressure. On the average, the students reported feelings of school pressure on five of the ten days sampled. So it would appear that such feelings were experienced by nearly all the students studied, and they seemed to arise frequently.

Another question in the diary asked the students about feelings of anxiety and their cause. School was not mentioned in the question in any way, but responses like the following were common: "Worrying about exams, classes, papers." "I didn't study enough for my exam." "Didn't know if I would have enough time to finish my term paper." "I have too much work and not enough time." "I feel as though I will never catch up with my course work."

In analyzing our data, we found that students who were experiencing academic stress reported higher levels of general anxiety. These students also reported more stress-related physical complaints, such as diarrhea, nausea, weakness and skin flare-ups. Students who reported they were feeling high levels of academic stress often reported they were feeling somewhat depressed. They experienced feelings of defeat and loneliness, and said they wanted to find help in dealing with their problems. They reported more instances in which such depressed feelings persisted all through the day. Academic pressures seem to contribute to depressed feelings. Depressed feelings, in turn, made it more difficult for the students to start work or concentrate effectively.

In our study, we noticed an interesting difference in the way male and female students responded to academic pressures. The young men who were experiencing academic stress tended to report more difficulties in their intepersonal relations. They found themselves acting defensively, being harder to get along with and often felt, and openly expressed, anger. It was almost as if these students were waving a red flag, saying "I'm in a lousy mood. Keep out of my way." This reaction was less apparent in the young women in our study who were experiencing academic stress. Like the adolescent girls we discussed in the previous chapter, these women seemed to have contained the tension within themselves. However, they reported a relatively high number of physical symptoms.

The general picture that emerged from our research is that many students were experiencing stress reactions to examinations and related academic pressures, often accompanied by mild to moderate levels of depressed mood. What we found in undergraduate students may be intensified in student training in graduate departments and professional schools such as law and medicine. Research has suggested that as many as one out of four medical students may be experiencing moderate to severe levels of depression.[18] Some of these depressed students drop out of medical school.

Stress is almost inevitable in modern life and indeed may have always been the case for humankind. No matter what the source of the stress, pressures from school, conflicts in human relationships, difficulties on one's job, major changes in life or an accumulation of daily pressures, there is a potential in many of us to be overwhelmed. The potential is particularly high in those people who have biological and psychological

---

[18]*See Clark & Zeldow (1988). The statistics are based on the Beck Depression Inventory. The peak of 25 percent was observed near the end of the second year of medical school.*

vulnerabilities toward depression. When a person is not able to cope adequately with stress, there is a heightened probability of a depressed reaction.

Understanding this relationship is important in trying to prevent depression. It is possible to place some limits on the amount of stress in our lives and to deal with stress situations more effectively when they do occur. I shall discuss these possibilities in the second part of the book.

BIBLIOGRAPHY

Benjaminsen, S. (1981). Stressful life events preceding the crest of neurotic depression. *Psychological Medicine,* 11, 369–78.

Billings, A. G.; Cronkite, R. C.; & Moos, R. H. (1983). Social-environmental factors in unipolar depression: Comparisons of depressed and nondepressed controls. *Journal of Abnormal Psychology,* 92, 119–33.

Billings, A. G., & Moos, R. H. (1984). Coping, stress, and social resources among adults with unipolar depression. *Journal of Personality and Social Psychology,* 46, 877–91.

Blumberg, S. R., & Hokanson, J. E. (1983). The effects of another person's response style on interpersonal behavior in depression. *Journal of Abnormal Psychology,* 92, 196–209.

Bowlby, J. (1980). *Loss: Sadness and depression (Attachment and Loss,* vol. 3). New York: Basic Books.

Clark, D. A.; Beck, A. T.; & Stewart, B. (1990). Cognitive specificity and positive-negative affectivity: Complementary or contradictory views on anxiety and depression? *Journal of Abnormal Psychology,* 99, 148–55.

Clark, D. C., & Zeldow, P. B. (1988). Vicissitudes of depressed mood during four years of medical school. *Journal of American Medical Association,* 260, 2521–28.

Cohen, S., & Wills, T. A. (1985). Stress, social support, and the buffering hypothesis. *Psychological Bulletin,* 98, 310–57.

Cohen, W. S. (1985). Health promotion in the workplace: A prescription for good health. *American Psychologist,* 40, 213–16.

Coyne, J. C. (1976). Depression and the response of others. *Journal of Abnormal Psychology,* 85, 186–93.

_____. (1985). Studying depressed person's interactions with strangers and spouses. *Journal of Abnormal Psychology,* 94, 231–32.

Coyne, J. C.; Aldwin, C.; & Lazarus, R. S. (1981). Depression and coping in stressful episodes. *Journal of Abnormal Psychology,* 90, 439–47.

Coyne, J. C.; Kessler, R. C.; Tal, M.; Turnbull, J.; Wortman, C. B.; & Greden, J. F. (1987).Living with a depressed person. *Journal of Consulting and Clinical Psychology,* 55, 347–52.

Dobson, K. S. (1985). The relationships between anxiety and depression. *Clinical Psychology Review,* 5, 307–24.

Feather, N. T., & Barber, J. G. (1983). Depressive reactions and unemployment. *Journal of Abnormal Psychology,* 92, 185–95.

Folkman, S., & Lazarus, R. S. (1986). Stress processes and depressive symptomatology. *Journal of Abnormal Psychology,* 95, 107–13.

Frank, E.; Turner, S. M.; & Duffy, B. (1979). Depressive symptoms in rape victims. *Journal of Affective Disorders,* 1, 269–77.

Freud, S. (1959). *Mourning and melancholia.* In *Collected Papers,* vol. 4, 152–70. New York: Basic Books.

Hautzinger, M.; Linden, M.; & Hoffman, N. (1982). Distressed couples with and without a depressed partner: An analysis of their verbal interaction. *Journal of Behavior Therapy and Experimental Psychiatry,* 13, 307–14.

Holahan, C. J., & Moos, R. H. (1991). Life stressors, personal and social resources, and depression: A four-year structural model. *Journal of Abnormal Psychology,* 100, 31–38.

Kanner, A. D.; Coyne, J. C.; Schaefer, C.; & Lazarus, R. S. (1981). Comparison of two modes of stress measurement: Daily hassles and uplifts versus major life events. *Journal of Behavioral Medicine,* 4, 1–39.

Kowalik, D. L., & Gotlib, I. H. (1987). Depression and marital interaction: Concordance between intent and perception of communication. *Journal of Abnormal Psychology,* 96, 127–34.

Leckman, J. F.; Merikangas, K. R.; Pauls, D. L.; Prusoff, B. A.; & Weissman, M. M. (1983). Anxiety disorders and depression: Contradictions between family study data and DSM-III conventions. *American Journal of Psychiatry,* 140, 880–82.

Lloyd, C. (1980). Life events and depressive disorder reviewed. II. Events as precipiating factors. *Archives of General Psychiatry,* 37, 541–48.

Maugham, W. S. (1955). *Of Human Bondage.* New York: Doubleday.

Meer, J. (1985, June). Blue-collar stress worse for boys. *Psychology Today,* 19, 15.

Meyersburg, H. A.; Ablon, S. L.; & Kotin, J. (1974). A reverberating psychic mechanism in the depressive processes. *Psychiatry,* 37, 372–86.

Murrell, S. A., & Himmelfarb, S. (1989). Effects of attachment bereavement and pre-event conditions on subsequent depressive symptoms in older adults. *Psychology and Aging,* 4, 166–72.

Robbins, P. R., & Tanck, R. H. (1984). Sex differences in problems related to depression. *Sex Roles,* 11, 703–7.

————, & ————. (1985, October 23). There are ways to fight college anxiety and stress. *Washington Post,* health section.

Roberts, M., & Harris, T. G. (1989, May). Wellness at work. *Psychology Today,* 54–58.

Shrout, P. E.; Link, B. G.; Dohrenwend, B. P.; Skodol, A. E.; Stueve, A.; & Mirotznik, J. (1989). Characterizing life events as risk factors for depression:

The role of fateful loss events. *Journal of Abnormal Psychology*, 98, 460–67.

Vaillant, G. E.; Sobowale, N. C.; and McArthur, C. (1972). Some psychological vulnerabilities of physicians. *New England Journal of Medicine*, 287, 372–75.

7. Depression, Alcohol and Drugs

Alcohol is a substance that has been used and abused since the development of urban civilization in ancient Mesopotamia. Archaeologists have unearthed metallic drinking straws dating back thousands of years, which may have been used for imbibing beer.

Today, the use of alcohol permeates our society, as well as many others. As Leif Crowe and William George put it, "Its consumption provides mystical trance, holy communion, celebration and consolation, social acceptance and condemnation, prowess and impotence, languor and lust. Indeed, there is scarcely a human activity that has not been said to be both impoverished and improved by the addition of alcohol."[1]

As we all know, alcohol abuse is a widespread problem. So, too, is drug abuse, which is now high on the agenda of our social problems. It has been estimated that five to ten million Americans are alcoholics.[2] Many more millions are alcohol abusers or have serious drinking problems. Moreover, millions of Americans use illegal drugs, some of which, like cocaine and heroin, are addictive.

If you talk with patients being treated for alcohol or drug addiction in hospital wards or in clinics, you will often find that these patients are or have been depressed. This is an important observation that has implications for the treatment and rehabilitation of substance abusers. In this chapter we will explore how depressed mood is linked to substance abuse.

[1]*Crowe & George (1989), p. 374.*
[2]*See National Institute of Alcohol Abuse and Alcoholism (1989).* Quick Facts *(revision May 8, 1989) estimated that the number of alcohol abusers and alcoholics in the United States would exceed 18,000,000 in 1990.*

Depression and Alcohol Abuse

Let us begin with alcoholism. Some years ago a noted authority on alcoholism wrote, "It is therefore a matter of clinical observation that preceding the use of alcohol there is always a depression."[3] While this assertion overstates the case, there is little doubt that in many people, depressed mood and the use of alcohol are linked. The linkage, however, is complicated.

On the one hand people may drink or use drugs as a way of relieving anxious and depressed moods. Alcohol and drugs are forms of self-medication: they make one feel better, at least temporarily. On the other hand, protracted substance use can lead to changes in life-style that can bring on depression. In this case the depression is considered secondary to the alcoholism.

To make the distinction between primary and secondary depression clearer, compare Eileen and Dan, two patients being treated for alcohol abuse. Eileen has had a plethora of emotional problems beginning in childhood. She experienced a rocky adolescence in which she had difficulties in getting along with her father, with her sexuality and in overcoming shyness. Both in her early childhood and teenage years, there were times in which she was withdrawn and very depressed.

Eileen's father and her father's family have a tradition of heavy drinking. When family members get together to eat or talk, there always seems to be an open bottle. Eileen joined in the family drinking in her teenage years and found that it made her feel better. She felt more confident and less tense. By the time she was out of college, she was a heavy, compulsive drinker who, in her own words, was "no longer drinking for fun" but because "she needed it." Drinking had become the preferred method of relieving tension and depression.

While Eileen's depressive problem preceded her alcoholism, Dan had no noticeable depressive problems until long after he began drinking. During high school Dan used "to party" with his friends. In his circle it was a matter of prestige to see how drunk you could get on weekends. The pattern of heavy drinking stayed with him after graduation and continued into his adult years. Drinking first cost him his job because of absenteeism and later his marriage. By the time he joined Alcoholics Anonymous (A.A.), he felt hopeless about his life, was filled with remorse

---

[3] *The assertion made by Benjamin Karpman is cited in Wall (1937).*

and guilt and was considering suicide. For Eileen, depression was primary to alcoholism. For Dan, depression was secondary to alcoholism. For some people depression precedes alcoholism and is intensified by it. Self-medicating only exacerbates the original problem.

Many alcoholic patients will report the usual symptoms of depression, ranging from poor sleep to feelings of hopelessness. A study carried out by David Clark and his colleagues suggests that the particular symptoms to look for in alcoholics, symptoms that point to depression, are guilt, self-disgust, irritability, indecision, dissatisfaction, work inhibition and loss of social interest.[4]

Just how strong is the tie-in between alcohol abuse and depression? If not all alcoholics are depressed, how many are? Many studies have been carried out on patients hospitalized for alcoholism. Sometimes these patients have been given psychiatric interviews using the *Diagnostic and Statistical Manual*'s criteria for depressive disorders. Sometimes they have been given self-report measures of depression. In reviewing these studies, David Lutz and Peggy Snow found that the estimates for depression among alcoholic patients varied considerably. Studies using the depression inventories suggest that a substantial majority of alcoholic patients are depressed. The figures from the psychiatric interviews do not seem quite as high but there are still estimates that exceed 50 percent. While it is not yet possible to offer a precise figure of the rate of depression among alcoholic patients, the numbers are substantial and may constitute a majority.

It is difficult to tell in how many of these persons' depression preceded the alcoholic problem and vice versa. To do so we usually have to depend on patients' memories about the past and we know that such memories can be faulty. It is interesting that when such studies are undertaken, the figures for depression preceding alcoholism run considerably higher for women than men. In studies cited in Lutz's and Snow's review, the figures for a preexisting depression in women were in the 25 percent range, while they were less than 10 percent for men.[5]

If these ballpark estimates — 10 to 25 percent — are approximately accurate, we would have to conclude that in most cases it is alcoholism that typically leads to depression, rather than the other way around.

[4]See *Clark et al (1985)*, pp. 483–85.

[5]See *Lutz's & Snow's (1985) review. These studies should be interpreted cautiously as the data are retrospective.*

While depression preceding alcoholism does not seem to be the typical pattern, it occurs often enough among women that it is certainly worth considering from a public health standpoint in terms of the prevention of alcoholism. The statistics suggest that alcohol has been adopted by a large number of women as a means of relieving depressed feelings. Therefore, one way of attacking the problem of alcoholism in women is to attack the causes of depression in women. The suggestion would be for society to deal more aggressively with the underlying problems that cause emotional difficulties in women rather than simply treating the symptoms of alcoholism.

When people are asked why they drink, or even more specifically, what effect they expect from drinking, they typically give the following answers: They expect to be more sociable, and to feel more relaxed and less inhibited. They also believe it will increase their enjoyment of sex.[6] They see some downside risks in drinking, such as acting foolishly or becoming aggressive, but in general they have a pretty rosy view of how they are going to feel after drinking. For people who are light to moderate drinkers, these expectations are often confirmed and this will sustain future drinking.

The problem comes when one is tempted to push the idea a little too far. If drinking can make one feel better and relieve the feelings of tension and pressure that have built up during the day, why not drink a little more and a little earlier? You'll feel better faster. And maybe alcohol will relieve the blue feelings we all experience at times when things go wrong and we are disappointed. These plausible ideas, unfortunately, lead one down the garden path.

There are several reasons for this. Heavy drinking throws one's normal intellectual and social abilities from order into chaos. One makes a mess out of what one is doing and one often ruins social relationships. Instead of increasing sexual enjoyment, heavy drinking often makes men impotent.[7] Heavy drinking leads one into dependency on alcohol. And alcohol is not particularly useful for relieving depression—other than blotting out reality entirely—for alcohol, itself, can have depressant effects.

People don't drink to feel more depressed, but that can happen, particularly for heavy drinkers. In a study carried out with alcoholics, the

---

[6]*For a discussion of expectations from drinking, see Brown et al. (1980).*
[7]*Crow & George (1989), p. 375.*

subjects were given adjective checklists to assess their moods before and after drinking. The scores for depressed mood were higher *after* drinking.[8] As alcohol can have depressant effects, it is of dubious value as an aid for coping with a depressed mood. Chances are that if alcohol is consumed in large amounts, it will only make matters worse. However, alcohol is inexpensive, available and people usually don't expect that to happen.

Secondary depression—the psychological effects of a deteriorating life-style that follows from prolonged alcohol use—may be a slow and insidious development, for the course of alcoholism itself is often protracted. Increasing dependence on alcohol doesn't happen overnight and one may exist with the problem for years before the roof finally caves in. By the time the person fully recognizes his or her alcoholic problems and enters a treatment program, a great deal of personal damage has accumulated. J. F. Nugent and I conducted a study of alcoholic patients at a Veterans Administration Hospital, in which we asked the patients whether their alcohol problem had caused any of a number of things to happen. We included the checklist of 17 items, which appears below. The percentage of the patients who responded yes are given in the column on the right.

Checklist Item	**Percentage Answering Yes**
1. Found it difficult to do my job well	49
2. Made me lose a job	38
3. Found myself in serious financial difficulties	54
4. Strained my relationship with members of my own family	73
5. Strained my relationship with my friends	43
6. Tried to conceal my using drugs from others	51
7. Got in trouble with the law	44
8. Spent time in jail	37
9. Stopped enjoying many of the things I used to enjoy	72
10. Began to find myself isolated	55
11. Found it difficult to concentrate	69

[8]*See Nathan et al. (1970).*

Checklist Item	Percentage Answering Yes
12. Began to feel tense and anxious	85
13. Began to have periods of depression	85
14. Had thoughts of suicide	27
15. Developed strong feelings of guilt about using drugs	78
16. Found I was living from day to day without planning for the future	67
17. Felt my life was in a downhill slide	75

As you can see from the percentages of patients who responded "yes, this problem happened to me," almost all of the patients had experienced tension and depression that they attributed to their alcohol problem. Psychologically, the patients felt that they were in a downhill slide. They felt guilty, aimless, were not enjoying their usual activities and felt increasingly isolated. All of these responses are consistent with a picture of depression. Typically, family relationships had been strained. Many of the patients had tried to conceal their problem from others. A sizeable number of the patients had experienced problems on their job, and over one-third of the patients had lost their jobs. Almost half of the patients reported having problems with the law and over a third had spent time in jail.

The depressing consequences of alcoholism emerge from these data. The real life stories that flesh out this skeleton of statistics may be heard over and over again at treatment centers and AA meetings. We also encounter such narratives in the psychology clinic. Following is an example showing the destructive interplay of depression and alcohol in the life of a young woman, Leila.

When Leila entered therapy at an outpatient clinic in San Francisco, she was recovering from alcoholism. She had been in AA for several years and had finally ceased drinking. As therapy began, Leila was tense. Her words were halting and measured and she was reticent in discussing many things that were still painful for her.

Leila was born in North Carolina and was raised by her mother, who had a chronic illness, and by her grandfather. Her father had been killed in an automobile accident when she was three years old. Her grandfather was a very strong person who raised her by the book and would tolerate no nonsense. Leila grew up to be a shy, passive person, used to being in the background. She did what she was told, though inwardly she felt resentful and spent as much time as she could away from her grandfather. In her school years she was something of a loner, never quite comfortable with the other children. Sometimes she felt lonely and rejected. The situation was only marginally improved when she went to college. She had no clear idea what she wanted to do, though she had some talent in painting and enjoyed her art classes.

In her final year of college, she met Frank. Frank was good looking, exceptionally bright, with an assertive dominating personality. Frank was the sort of person who would "take over." He was attracted to her physically, swept her off her feet and they were married shortly before graduation. Leila and Frank settled in a rather isolated community in southwestern Texas. Frank was busy with his job and Leila found herself alone a good deal of the time. This is when she began to drink.

Early on Frank began to show evidence of boredom with the marriage. He began to dwell on the intellectual discrepancy between himself and his wife, and became sarcastic when she made a mistake or showed ignorance on a subject. Leila became increasingly tense in their conversations. She felt cowed; it seemed almost like a replay of her childhood days with her grandfather. The more tense she became, the more she drank.

When their daughter, Charlotte, was born, Leila and Frank began to get along better, at least for a while. They moved first to Denver and then to San Francisco, where Frank's job put him into contact with many interesting people. Leila remained at home with Charlotte. Frank grew intellectually, Leila didn't. In time, Frank's sarcasm returned, now growing into contempt. He frequently put her down. Leila became unsettled emotionally. She felt trapped, tense and depressed. She drank heavily.

Alcohol gave her courage. She got into bloody arguments with her husband, often in front of her young daughter. However, Leila was no match for him when sober, and alcohol only dulled her wits. She became incoherent, angry and emotionally out of control. Frank reacted by leaving home for days at a time and became involved with several women. Finally he left altogether and filed for divorce.

When the marriage was shattered, Leila found herself with few resources, an alcohol problem and depression. She tried making it on her own, but lacked confidence and was drinking too much. She couldn't hold a job. She had difficulty making new friends and felt isolated. She contemplated suicide and for a while was hospitalized.

Alcoholics Anonymous helped her turn things around. In therapy she began to explore her own needs and to develop a more positive sense of her own identity. In therapy, the focus in her life changed for the first time to what she could do for herself and what she could become. She was able to get a job and to begin to build a life of her own.

Depression and Illegal Drugs

Let's talk about illegal drugs—the black market drugs that are sold on the street. One of the most widely used of the illegal drugs, marijuana, has certain pharmacological depressant effects. Research has been carried out on a variety of animals—squirrels, monkeys, cats and rats—looking at the effect of the drug on activity level. Interestingly, the effect of the drug is often biphasic; i.e., there is an initial period of excitement and stimulation, which is followed by quiet behavior in which the animals move about less and do little.[9] Similar effects have been reported with human subjects. Many people become sleepy after using marijuana and report a decline in activity.

People use marijuana because of the anticipated effects of the drug. They expect a "high" from the drug and to feel relaxed. They usually hope to attain these pleasant moods in the company of friends. Smokers report such sensations as lightheadedness, giddiness, intensified perception such as seeing colors more intensely, sexual arousal, dryness in the mouth, hunger and sleepiness. Adverse effects from the drug are not usual, but happen often enough to be of concern. Users of the drug at times experience feelings of anxiety and depression. In one study, 40 percent of the users questioned reported that they had experienced such reactions.[10]

The person who has used marijuana on an occasional, recreational basis is unlikely to have concomitant emotional problems more than nonusers. The situation changes, however, when marijuana use becomes frequent and it becomes a stepping stone into the world of harder drugs. A life-style in which illegal drugs becomes a centerpiece carries with it increased risk of psychological problems. As with alcoholism, it can be difficult to distinguish between preexisting personality tendencies that

[9]*Robbins (1983), p. 27.*
[10]*See Keeler et al. (1971).*

lead to the use of drugs and the emotional wreckage that often results from drug addiction.

Perhaps the best illustration of the difficulties caused by drug abuse are the stories of heroin addicts. Heroin is often the end-of-the-line drug when everything else has been tried. Heroin was originally developed with the best of intentions, as a "nonaddictive substitute" for morphine, which was in medical use as a painkiller. The problem was that heroin turned out to be highly addictive, producing both tolerance (you don't get as much effect from the drug if you keep using it, so you have to step up the dose to get the same effect) and physical dependence (you need to keep using the drug the prevent the beginning of uncomfortable withdrawal symptoms).

Heroin is a very potent pain reliever. Unlike marijuana, which may be associated with increased sexual arousal, heroin use may decrease sexual interest. The drug may have an uplifting effect on many people, can act as a tranquilizer for tension, and may detach the individual from the realities of the day.[11] Life may take on a rosy hue until the effect of the drug wears off. It is this euphoric effect that draws many people to the drug.

When a person becomes physically addicted to heroin and stops using it, withdrawal symptoms occur. Such symptoms may include nausea, diarrhea, vomiting, abdominal cramps, profuse sweating, nervousness and insomnia. Symptoms usually diminish within a few days, but a craving for heroin may persist for years. This craving often leads to resumption of use.

Dependence on a drug such as heroin can become overwhelming. Some people who are addicted to this drug may do almost anything to again experience the sensations that they remember from past use of the drug. They will put aside all the other memories—the misery that drug abuse has caused them in their lives—to experience the drug sensation. Hard drugs can exert a fatal attraction that reminds one of the story of the Sirens in the *Odyssey*, in which the song of these nymphs lured sailors to their deaths as their ships smashed on the rocks.

The psychological and social destruction of the heroin addict is similar in many ways to that of the alcoholic. The main difference is that it is usually quicker. There are reasons for this precipitous decline. Heroin use causes a physical addiction that requires continued use of the

[11]*See National Clearinghouse for Drug Abuse Information (1975), p. 9.*

drug to prevent withdrawal symptoms. Unlike alcohol, which is also addictive, heroin is expensive and to sustain this drug habit costs a bundle. The victim soon has an empty pocketbook and often is induced into illegal activities, such as robbery or selling drugs, to buy more drugs. The chances of being arrested are pretty high.

Take a second look at the list of consequences we used in our research with alcoholics. We gave the list with the same instructions to two samples of patients under treatment for heroin addiction. One group of patients was hospitalized, undergoing detoxification and therapy. The other group of patients was being treated on an outpatient basis; most were on methadone maintenance. Some statistics from our study showed that the inpatients in particular had encountered very serious financial and legal problems as a consequence of drug dependency. Eight-five percent of the hospitalized patients reported they had experienced serious financial difficulties. Eight-two percent had gotten into trouble with the law. Sixty-seven percent had spent time in jail. The psychological consequences of addiction for these inpatients were also severe. Ninety-seven percent of the patients reported they had periods of depression. Ninety-four percent felt their lives were on a downhill slide. Eighteight percent reported they were becoming isolated. Forty-two percent had thoughts of suicide.

As we can see from these data, almost all of the inpatients in the study indicated that depression was one of the consequences of heroin addiction. From interviews we conducted with other heroin-addicted patients, however, I have the impression that for many people who use heroin, depressive tendencies had set in earlier in life and were intensified by the life-style of the heroin addict.

Many of the patients interviewed had experienced a childhood and adolescence that nurtured a depressive outlook.[12] A large number of the patients had come from homes in which there was no father present, or, perhaps worse, a father who was alcoholic, indifferent or abusive. We know from research on child development that such circumstances increase the chances of depressive problems. The experience of school for many was not helpful and the jobs that were available tended to be boring and dead-end.

A growing sense of futility opened the way for drug experimentation. To many, it seemed as if there was little going for them and little to hope

---

[12]*For further discussions of these data, see Robbins (1974).*

for—so why not go for some kicks in life? Most of the patients felt that
—they would not become addicted; there was a sense of invulnerability—
"It won't happen to me." The consequences of addiction, however, often
proved devastating, resulting in severe depressive problems. Almost all
the studies that I have seen found elevated levels of depression among
inpatients being treated for heroin addiction.

Drug addiction often leads to a kind of twilight existence. Addicts
move surreptitiously in circles of other addicts and pushers. Many of
them conceal what they are doing from their families as long as they can
but the unrelenting need for the drug usually leads to family strains and
financial disaster. The resulting conflict and misery can be glimpsed in
excerpts from statements of the addicts themselves.

> "I feel very depressed. I was unhappy with being out of work, out of money,
> being drug addicted. Using drugs has hurt my self-confidence. I feel I have
> messed up so many times in the past, I will do it again in the future."
>
> "My wife got ready to leave me. I attempted suicide."
>
> "I feel super depressed. Things piling up, bills, family things—makes me
> worried and depressed. Life on drugs made me go through more hell and
> frustration and more sickness than it's [possible] to imagine."
>
> "I couldn't trust myself when I was strung out."
>
> "The problem has been a constant struggle for my wife . . . I get disgusted
> at myself in preparation stage, but once I am high, I don't give a damn."
>
> "I felt I was going down, down, down. I had to get off of it."
>
> "Living the life of an addict is really hell. After you've become hooked it's
> pure hell. An addict may be smiling on the outside—but inside he's crying—
> it's a thing that bites and bites."

BIBLIOGRAPHY

Blatt, S. J.; McDonald, C.; Sugarman, A.; & Wilber, C. (1984). Psychodynamic
theories of opiate addiction: New directions for research. *Clinical
Psychology Review*, 4, 159–89.

Bowden, C. L. (1971). Determinants of initial use of opioids. *Comprehensive
Psychiatry*, 12, 136–40.

Brown, S. A.; Goldman, M. S.; Inn, A.; & Anderson, L. R. (1980). Expectations
of reinforcement from alcohol: Their domain and relation to drinking patterns. *Journal of Consulting and Clinical Psychology*, 48, 419–26.

Clark, D. C.; Gibbons, R. D.; Fawcett, J.; Aagesen, C. A.; & Sellers, D. (1985).
Unbiased criteria for severity of depression in alcoholic inpatients. *Journal
of Nervous and Mental Disease*, 173, 482–87.

Crowe, L. C., & George, W. H. (1989) Alcohol and human sexuality: Review and integration. *Psychological Bulletin*, 105, 374–86.

Keeler, M. H.; Ewing, J. A.; & Rouse, B. A. (1971). Hallucinogenic effects of marijuana as currently used. *American Journal of Psychiatry*, 128, 213–16.

Keeler, M. H.; Taylor, C. I.; & Miller, W. C. (1979). Are all recently detoxified alcoholics depressed? *American Journal of Psychiatry*, 136, 586–88.

Lutz, D. J., & Snow, P. A. (1985). Understanding the role of depression in the alcoholic. *Clinical Psychology Review*, 5, 535–51.

Nathan, P. E.; Titler, N. A.; Lowenstein, L. M.; Solomon, P.; & Rossie, A. M. (1970). Behavioral analysis of chronic alcoholism. *Archives of General Psychiatry*, 22, 419–30.

National Clearinghouse for Drug Abuse Information (1975). *Heroin*. Series 33, no. 1. DHEW publication no. (ADM) 74-198.

National Institute of Alcohol Abuse and Alcoholism (1989). *Quick facts*. Revised ed. Rockville, Md.: Author.

Robbins, P. R. (1974). Depression and drug addiction. *Psychiatric Quarterly*, 48, 374–86.

_____ (1974). *Problems and treatment of heroin addiction in the United States*. Leonia, N.J.: Sigma Information, Behavioral Science Tape Library.

_____ (1983). *Marijuana: A short course. Update for the eighties*. Brookline Village, Mass.: Branden.

_____, & Nugent J. F., III. (1975). Perceived consequences of addiction: A comparison between alcoholics and heroin-addicted patients. *Journal of Clinical Psychology*, 31, 367–69.

Wall, J. H. (1937). A study of alcoholism in women. *American Journal of Psychiatry*, 93, 942–55.

Weissman, M. M., & Myers, J. K. (1980). Clinical depression in alcoholism. *American Journal of Psychiatry*, 137, 372–73.

Winokur, G.; Reich, T.; Rimmer, J.; & Pitts, F. N., Jr. (1970). Alcoholism: III. Diagnosis and familial psychiatric illness in 259 alcoholic probands. *Archives of General Psychiatry*, 23, 104–11.

8. Coping with Depressed Feelings

Now that we have completed our inquiry into the nature of depressed moods and states, it is time to ask what you can do about them. What steps can you take to prevent depression? How can you cope with depressed feelings when they occur? In addressing these questions, we are going to first look at what a person can do to deal with his or her own depressed feelings. Then we will look at the way family and friends can help. Finally, we will look at what mental health professionals may offer in the way of medicine, psychotherapy and other treatments.

When we discuss self-help in preventing depression, we are largely talking about gaining increased control over your life. To move in this direction may require both changes in thought patterns or mind-sets and changes in behavior. In this process you should begin to view life in more positive terms, to recognize that you can bring changes into your life, and that your efforts can make a difference in the way you feel.

Setting Rewarding and Reachable Goals

In looking at some of the ways you can gain more control over your life, let's begin with the question of setting rewarding, yet reachable goals. Consider these questions: Do you have goals for the near future—for the next weeks or months? Do you have longer range goals—for the years ahead? Take a few moments and try spelling out what you would like to accomplish, both in the near term and in the more distant future. Now consider if these are reasonable goals, things that you have a decent chance of achieving. If they are, fine. But if they seem unrealistic, where does that leave you? You may be setting yourself up for more failure and

117

disappointment, which may lead to the question "What's wrong with me?" The result may be a further erosion of self-esteem.

A woman came to see me in therapy. She was 45 years old. She had average ability. Her college grades had been mostly Cs. She told me she was thinking about applying to law school. Realistically, the chances are she would have a hard time both getting into and through a law school and would be pushing 50 if and when she got her degree. Further, it is questionable how competitive she would be in the job market at that point. One doesn't like to discourage aspirations, but if she had chosen a more attainable goal, it would have increased the chances of her experiencing success rather than disappointment.

There is a wonderful song in the musical *The Man of La Mancha* called "The Impossible Dream." You may remember both the song and the play, based upon Cervantes's story of Don Quixote. The lyrics of the song speak about reaching unreachable goals. Now, there are people who are made of sturdy enough stuff to try this, who can tolerate endless frustrations in the search of deeply rooted ambitions. One thinks of artists like Van Gogh, who painted masterpieces that no one would buy, actors who lived from hand-to-mouth while trying to make it on the stage or the minor league baseball player who couldn't make it into the big leagues, but never quit trying.

I have always encouraged patients who believe that they have the talent to do something to go ahead and give their dreams their best shot so they will not spend life wondering what they might have been. But I also advise them to keep a dash of realism—not to end up tilting at windmills like Don Quixote.

While unrealistic goals can lead to disappointment and depressed reactions, setting goals that are very low, unchallenging and raise little risk, can also lead to a life of frustration and unrealized potential. A life of self-selected mediocrity can be bitter and depressing.

There are, of course, many reasons that prevent people from doing things that challenge them and afford them the opportunity to develop their full potential. Job openings may not be available. The person may lack education or economic resources, or be burdened by heavy responsibilities for the care of family members. However, for many people, selecting a restrictive life-style is a result of psychological factors. Fear of failure and taking risks has kept many people locked into situations that offer little fulfillment. The result is often dependency, frustration and depressed mood.

Goal setting that is unrealistic on the one side or unchallenging on the other raises the potential for problems. Ideally, when we set goals, we would like them to be desirable, challenging, yet attainable. It should be not only what we want to achieve, but the sort of things that our talents, resources and personal characteristics give us a reasonable chance of bringing to fruition.

Clearly, self-analysis is required in goal setting. There are important questions to consider. What are the things you really want? What things do you do best? What are your weaknesses? Do you have the patience and persistence necessary to follow through to achieve what you want? Do you have problems like fear of failure or difficulties in asserting yourself that might intefere with reaching your goals? If such issues are troublesome for you, perhaps you may want to discuss them with a counselor or therapist.

Analysis of the goals themselves and what is necessary to achieve them is also important. Consider career decisions as an example. Do you know the kinds of training that are necessary to get into the type of work that you would like to do? Do you know what future job opportunities are likely to exist in this line of work?

When you think about career goals, you might want to research such questions. It may be helpful to talk to people who are working in the field. Also, look over the resources in the public library. Ask the librarian for *The Occupational Outlook Handbook,* put out by the Department of Labor. It's loaded with information. If you are unsure about your aptitudes and interests, you may find it useful to call the counseling center at your local college or university. They may offer vocational counseling and have interesting tests to help you more objectively evaluate yourself.

Taking a Look at Where You Are

If you have been feeling depressed, chances are that you could profit from making a general reassessment of what's going on in your life. In doing so, you might find it helpful to talk things over with someone who you have confidence in—someone who can react to your ideas and offer another perspective. Consider a minister, a counselor, a therapist— someone who you trust and feel comfortable with. Listening to the reactions of another person is helpful for most people and may be particularly important if you are prone to depression, for depression often gives you a negative bias in looking at yourself and the world about you.

The idea in this assessment is to identify what is going right in your life and what is not. Ask yourself what things bring satisfaction to your life and what are sources of stress and unhappiness. This task is something like taking personal inventory, but it is also a beginning of diagnosis. Your objective is to determine where it is desirable to make changes in what you are doing.

Be specific in your thinking. If you say, "I don't like my job," it may be that there are only *some aspects* of your job you don't like. Perhaps it is a co-worker who is giving you a problem or it may be one of your duties that you particularly dislike. When you pinpoint things, it is easier to discuss making possible changes. Remember, people who get depressed have a tendency to overgeneralize. The fact that there are some problems does not mean everything is bad.

Frequently the problem that is upsetting you will be in human relationships. For example, you may find yourself in a situation where you care a great deal about another person, but there are things about that person that you find irritating. Ambivalence—having both positive and negative feelings toward another person—is part of the human experience. Can you pinpoint the negatives, the things that are bothering you? Is it possible that something could be done to make the situation more livable?

In pinpointing the things that are upsetting you—the situations that are creating stress in your life—you may look at your environment (your home life, your place of work, your relationships) and you may also look at yourself. Are you doing things now that you would like to be doing differently? Ask yourself, where would you like to see changes in yourself?

Changing Patterns of Thinking

When we talk about changes, we include both changes in thought patterns or mind-sets and changes in behavior. Sometimes just looking at situations differently can make a difference in whether you are likely to feel depressed.

I have discussed research that indicates that the way a person evaluates a situation makes a difference. If you tend to inflate the importance of events, to magnify what is at stake, then you may be setting yourself up for an overreaction. The trick is to be able to distinguish between what is *really important* and what is *not*. If you act as if everything falls in the former category, then be prepared to ride on an emotional roller coaster and have your self-esteem beaten down like a rug at spring cleaning. When you sense you are about to get riled up over something that is trivial, stop and ask yourself, "What am I doing?" Surely there are enough important things in your life to be concerned about without going bonkers over things that don't really matter.

A woman with a teenaged son developed an acrimonious relationship with him, putting both of them under a lot of unnecessary stress by making repeated issues out of such things as the way he decorated his room with rock star posters, the way he dressed and the way he sometimes procrastinated in doing chores like mowing the lawn. The relationship would have been a lot smoother had she acknowledged that the important things in his life were going well—he got good grades in school, stayed clear of drugs and had many friends. What the mother needed was a larger measure of tolerance, an understanding that other people can do things in a different manner from you and the world will not fall apart.

I have also mentioned being hung up on comparisons with other people as a thinking pattern that promotes depression. One of my favorite examples of these comparison traps is a patient who came to see me who was the operator of a photocopy business. The man had practically no formal education. He worked very hard in his business, putting in long hours, and made an excellent income. I thought he had done very well, having started and successfully run a small business. When I ventured this opinion to him, he shook his head forlornly and replied that he was a failure. In explaining his feelings, he told me about a man who had a similar business three blocks away. It was a larger, more attractive shop that offered more services and had more machines. The other shop was doing more business and making more money than my patient's shop and he felt demoralized by this.

We grow up in a world of comparisons. We are defined by others as being bigger or smaller or smarter or not so smart or more attractive or less attractive, and so on. While such comparisons are inevitable in the way we are raised, it does not mean that we have to orient our adult thinking and lives this way. There is an alternative approach. This approach is to carefully define your own goals—goals that are desirable and attainable for yourself—and go after them. The measure of your success is the extent to which you attain your goals. What other people decide to seek in life is their concern, and need not be a gauge for your own evaluation of success.

If you measure yourself against what everyone else is doing, it's almost impossible to win. If you have your own goals in life and meet them, you can feel you are doing what you want and can experience a sense of satisfaction. It's all in the way you define success. My patient's attitude was self-defeating. Even if he had owned the larger of the two photocopy shops, there would always be someone else who had a larger one.

In discussing thinking patterns that need changing, let's recall another source of difficulty: perfectionist thinking. Do you have this tendency? Here are a few signs:

> You are chronically dissatisfied.
> Nothing is ever good enough to please you.
> Things have to be ordered just so—nothing can be out of place.
> Everything has to be done on time.
> Your house and yard must look like a museum.
> You find faults with everybody.
> You obsess about the quality of your work.
> You seldom finish anything because "it isn't good enough."
> Your motto is, "Don't do anything unless you can do it right."
> People tell you that you are a nitpicker.

If you find yourself nodding your head and saying, "That's me, all right," you have a problem.[1] What can you do about it? As a beginning, try to recognize these patterns in your thoughts and behavior when they occur. Recognition of your tendency toward perfectionism is an important step in doing something about it. Then take a good look at your behavior, or better yet, what such behavior is doing to you and the other people in your life. As you reflect on this, you will probably find that standards of perfectionism are interfering with your ability to get things done and with your feelings of satisfaction from what you are doing. It is also turning off other people and causing them problems.

This may be a hard idea to accept and you could be inclined to argue

---

[1]*Paul Hewitt and Gordon Flett have developed a reliable scale to measure perfectionist tendencies. See Hewitt & Flett (1991).*

"Well, isn't it important to do things well?" The answer is sure. Making a solid effort and turning out high-quality work are very important values. To be hung up on an error-free existence, however, is something else, a burden one would not wish on anyone. If you are a perfectionist, loosen the screws on yourself and others. Try being more tolerant and less critical. See if you and everyone else are not a little more relaxed and a lot happier as a result.

Reinforce Yourself Instead of Kicking Yourself

We could title this section, "give yourself a break." Many people who become depressed are much more inclined to get down on themselves for making mistakes than to pat themselves on the back for doing something well. It is something like a football game where the fans boo when you fumble the ball but don't cheer when you score a touchdown. Consider this: positive reinforcement builds up self-esteem, nonconstructive criticism tears it down.

When you do something well, tell yourself you "did OK." When you accomplish something that you've wanted to do, smile and give yourself some credit. When you've done something especially satisfying, how about going out and celebrating? Do something you really like or buy something you've always wanted. How about that new sweater or jacket? It will help you move away from the idea that life is nothing but a series of negatives.

Reinforcing yourself is one of the ways of moving toward a more optimistic perspective about your life. Another mind-set that will help nudge you in this direction is to give yourself the benefit of the doubt when something goes wrong. When things go awry, too often depression-prone people look inwardly and stop there. The conclusion may be almost automatic, "It's my fault."

The conclusion may be true, it may be partly true or it may not be true at all. We live in a complex world where cause and effect is seldom very clear. How many things are *totally* under your control? Not many, if you think about it. You depend on other people to do things in a very interrelated society. When someone else fails to come through, it may affect your ability to do what you're trying to do. What do you do when someone else screws up? Or consider all the uncontrollables in life. Can you control traffic, the weather, catching a virus, your boss's temperament, the state of the job market? If something goes wrong, there may be some very good reasons for what happened besides something you did. Let's suppose you did make a mistake on something. Before overreacting and lapsing into a sea of gloom, ask yourself these questions: Do you know anyone who doesn't make mistakes? Is the mistake you made catastrophic? The answer is likely to be no to both questions. So, pick up the pieces and move on.

When you do have negative experiences, it is vital that you do not overgeneralize. As we have indicated, many people who become depressed have a tendency to turn negative experiences into calamities. In contrast, the person who remains emotionally intact often finds a way to shrug it off. Her reaction may be, "c'est la vie," or "so what?" She limits the impact. She does not get down on herself; rather, she searches for the next opportunity, recognizing that success is likely to come only if she keeps trying. The person who resists depression may not only brush aside the negative experience but downgrade its importance. Defense mechanisms rationalize failures away. This may seem unrealistic, but it offers protection. While you may not always be able to put the best face on a negative experience, to avoid becoming depressed try not to put the worst face on it. It helps if you keep your sense of perspective and don't overgeneralize.

Changes in Behavior

Changing attitudes and thought patterns are important steps in protecting oneself against the onset of depressive episodes. Equally important are changes in behavior. In your assessment of things that you would like to do differently, you probably spelled out some specific changes you would like to make. Let's talk about getting started.

One way of approaching change is to adopt a strategy of small wins.[2] This strategy recognizes that you can't do everything at once, and to try too much too soon can set you up for more experience of failure. If you've been depressed, you don't need any more of that. In a strategy of small wins, you begin with a defined goal and start taking steps toward realizing it. When you've taken a step in the right direction and experienced some success—"a small win"—reinforce yourself.

[2]*The strategies of small wins is discussed by Weick (1984).*

A woman who was feeling depressed came to see me. She reported that one of her biggest problems was feeling lonely. Too many nights she had nothing to do and no one to see. The weekends were particularly depressing. After a few therapy sessions, she agreed to join a club where she would have an opportunity to meet people. Finding out about clubs and organizations that might interest her was an important first step. She did this by looking through the notices posted at her public library. As she was an outdoors-type person, she chose a local hiking club that went on outings on the weekends. She called the number listed on the notice and with some anxiety attended her first meeting. She found that the people were nice and she enjoyed the walks. On her third outing, she met an interesting man and began dating him. She wasn't sure whether the relationship would pan out, but she is making friends and her loneliness is fading. My patient told me that at each step toward becoming more involved in the club, she felt a little anxious. There is a certain amount of risk involved in starting new undertakings. But risk taking is necessary if you are going to make changes. And if you are depressed, changes are usually necessary.

A careful, step-by-step approach minimizes risks and anxiety that might be aroused. A strategy of small wins builds confidence and provides the opportunity for larger successes. My patient who joined the hiking club experienced some stress in the process of becoming a member and making friends. Going through this discomfort was necessary to attain an important objective—dealing with her loneliness. Many people who are prone to depression already have too many stressors in their lives, stressors they can't handle, so care and timing are important when a person who is depressed contemplates adding new activities. But these steps are important as they can rebuild confidence and rekindle hope, both of which are important psychological medicines against depression. A poet once put it well, "Each forward step we take we leave some phantom of ourselves behind."[3]

Overcoming Resistance to Change

Change is sometimes a difficult thing to bring about. You'll often find resistance to making needed changes both in yourself and in others. I

[3]*This line was attributed to J. L. Spaulding.*

mentioned that change involves taking risks. The anticipation of risks elicits anxiety, and anxiety can be very uncomfortable. An all-too-easy way to terminate anxiety is to call a halt to what you are planning to do. Of course, that leaves you right where you started from, in a malaise.

You might use rationalizations to prop up a decision not to carry your plan through. Can you hear the inner voice, "I didn't really want to do that anyway. Besides, it wouldn't have worked." People who are depressed often have a negative perspective and it is very easy to convince themselves that anything they try won't work. After all, hasn't their history been one of failure? Why should they expect anything different?

It can be very hard to break through a demoralized attitude. Some encouragement from family and friends can be helpful and so can the actions of an energizing therapist. Still, the bottom line comes down to the person who is feeling depressed. If you want to feel better, you have to start doing things. Reading books such as this is an indication that you want to make changes and is a positive sign that you can. Beginning steps, small wins and confidence building are the orders of the day.

Many of the sources of stress that make life difficult involve our relationships with other people. Stress on the job often involves your relationship with your boss or conflicts with other employees. Stress in the home life usually involves other people. And stress in romantic relationships can be an important, and at times, overwhelming concern.

To make changes in the way people interact can be a difficult undertaking. When you express the wish to introduce changes in a relationship, the idea that is generated is "something is wrong." And if you do not handle the situation adroitly, the other person may then think, "You're accusing me of doing something wrong." This notion can trigger an emotional reaction of defensiveness. You may encounter hurt feelings, avoidance, the silent treatment or indignation. One can almost hear the denials. "I did not! I am not!" The anger that is provoked may lead to retaliation. "You're the one who is at fault." The attempt to reduce stress has only resulted in increased levels of stress.

The possibility of this all-too-familiar scenario is enough to discourage many people from even trying to suggest changes. However, if the current situation is making life unlivable, you have little choice but to try. Diplomacy is often the best bet. One approach is to say something like this: "You know, I've been under a lot of stress. I've been feeling bad and I'm trying to make a few changes. Can you help me?" In this context, it makes it a little harder to refuse.

One of the ways to lower resistance in others is to ask for their input, their ideas. If some of the things they suggest make sense to you, incorporate these ideas into an overall package that includes your own ideas. Propose the overall package as a joint plan and see if you and the other party or parties can agree to the plan. A process like this where everyone's ideas are considered seriously, and where an agreement can be reached, has added force and staying power.

Many people who become depressed have problems in asserting themselves, in making known what they want to do and what they don't want to do. Such people often have a hard time in saying no. This reluctance to communicate their true wishes adds to the difficulty of making needed changes. The alternative of not speaking up, of accepting a bad situation, of course, merely prolongs the situation that led to the depressed reaction.

There are books, even courses, on assertiveness training. The goal of assertiveness training is usually to learn how to state your wishes in a clear, convincing manner without being argumentative, and if you don't want to do something, you practice saying no. You learn how to give a simple reason for your decision without becoming bogged down in lengthy explanations, which may only weaken your case. Being able to be assertive when you need to be is an important tool is making the kind of changes you wish to make. If you have a problem being assertive, it is a skill you can learn.

Start with Exercise

When people come to see me and tell me that they are feeling depressed, one of the first things I often recommend is that they start an exercise program. I always ask them to check with their doctors first to be clear about their physical condition and to find out what level of exercise is safe and appropriate, what is well within their capabilities.

Within these guidelines, I don't think it really matters very much what type of exercise you choose, whether it's tennis, riding an indoor bicycle or walking. The latter is usually a safe and satisfying way to begin. Imagine a daily routine that includes a pleasant walk in the park, or along city streets with interesting shops and lots of people, or perhaps a tree-lined suburban road. Some people find that just being in a pleasant setting, enjoying the beauties of the natural world is therapeutic. The poet

John Keats wrote about immersing oneself in nature when downcast. In his poem, *Ode on Melancholy*, he wrote,

> But when the melancholy fit shall fall
>   Sudden from heaven like a weeping cloud,
> That fosters the droop-headed flowers all,
>   And hides the green hills in an April shroud;
> Then glut thy sorrow on a morning rose,
>   Or on the rainbow of the salt sand-wave,
>   Or on the wealth of globed peonies...

Whether it is a park, a suburban road, or a modern health spa—whatever you prefer as a setting—find a place that's safe and pleasant, then *move*. In a word, exercise is the thing!

The reason I suggest starting an exercise program as a first step in combating depressed feelings is that there is considerable research evidence that indicates that exercise has an antidepressive effect.[4] Some of the reasons for this effect may be physiological, but there are important psychological benefits as well. Among the psychological effects is the fact that you can see that you are accomplishing something and you will make measurable progress in accomplishing more. For example, if you are riding an indoor bicycle, you can ride increasingly longer distances. This can give you a psychological lift. Exercise is a good way to reduce tension. Moreover, exercise tones you up. You feel better, you look better, your wind and stamina are better. You feel more alive.

When you select an exercise program, it is important to choose something you really like to do. Don't start a regimen of doing sit-ups if you hate sit-ups. A pleasant routine of exercise is most likely to be antidepressant.

Look Better, Feel Better

Exercise may help you look better, and for many people, that in itself may make them feel better. Studies have shown that people who feel better about their appearance tend to have brighter psychological outlooks.

[4]*See Simons et al. (1985).*

This is particularly true for adolescents and young adults where appearance is often highly valued.[5]

It is certainly true that if one is pleased about the way one looks, it can help one's confidence and self-esteem. For many people, shaping up to look better can be part of an overall therapeutic plan of behavioral change to cope with depressed feelings. Shaping up may include weight loss, if weight is a problem, and toning up one's body.

Dietary changes might be considered along with appropriate exercise. It is quite possible that dietary changes in and of themselves may have antianxiety and antidepressant effects.[6] Research has suggested, for example, that excessive use of caffeine may be associated with anxiety in some people.[7] If you live on coffee and have been feeling tense, try a substitute and see if it helps.

Recalling Wurtman's research on diet, some people with serotonin deficiencies may have accidentally discovered that eating high carbohydrate, low-protein meals improves their mood because such foods increase serotonin synthesis. People with low levels of serotonin who have become carbohydrate snackers are in a sense medicating themselves. Snacking on carbohydrates could become a habit for such people if it makes them feel better.

Some therapists have suggested to their depressed patients to consider buying new clothes.[8] For many people, an attractive wardrobe has a place in looking better and feeling better about oneself.

> Mirror, mirror on the wall.
> Who is looking better these days?
> C'est moi!

[5]See *Cash et al. (1986)* and the recent work of *Betty Allgood-Merten et al (1990)*. In discussing their research on adolescence, Allgood-Merten and her colleagues state, "The results also corroborate the finding that body image is an important correlate of depression in adolescence. . . . [Body image] is a critically important aspect of self-esteem in this age group that functions as an antecedent as well as a strong correlate of depressive symptoms in adolescents." Allgood-Merten et al. (1990), p. 61.

[6]*Larry Christensen and Ross Burrows* conducted an experiment in which ten depressed persons were instructed to eliminate caffeine and refined sucrose from their diet. These persons were compared with ten depressed patients who were put on a control diet. Using depression scales such as the BDI as criteria, the investigators found that the subjects who eliminated caffeine and refined sucrose reported lower levels of depression. See Christensen & Burrows (1990).

[7]See *Veleber and Templer (1984)*.

[8]See *Solomon (1986)*.

Introduction of Pleasant Activities

Could you list five or six activities you really enjoy? Taking walks, going to the movies, swimming, going to a party, listening to music, whatever. Take a few minutes and come up with your own list. All right, how many of these things are you doing now? If you're not doing some of these things, wouldn't it make sense to start? A life with no fun is depressing.

In planning changes in your life, see if it is possible to give a higher priority to these activities. If you can, you will probably find that this will cause a shift in the negative-positive balance in your daily life. You will have more things to look forward to and this is likely to elevate your mood.[9]

In thinking about this idea, try not to put it into a "must-do" framework. These activities should be things you *want to do,* not things you feel you have to do. Viewing such activities as ordered or imposed will only take the joy out of them. Just start doing some of the things you've always liked doing and do them at a pace you find right for you.

Developing Meaningful Social Relationships

Much of what is meaningful and important in life is having friends and loved ones, feeling a sense of inter-connectedness with other people. Many people who report depressed feelings feel lonely. They don't have many friends; they often feel isolated. When things go well, they may not have people with whom to share their good tidings. When things go badly, they may have no one to reach out to. If this is the case, it is important to try to do something about it. Having close friends is an important element in preventing depressed reactions. Good friends act as a buffer in times of stress.

A typical problem that one hears from depressed people is "How do I meet people? How do I make new friends?" It's not always easy to do this when you're young and in school and it probably doesn't get any easier as you find yourself separated from the people you grew up with

[9]*A study reported by Douglas Needles and Lyn Abramson suggested that the introduction of pleasant activities into one's daily life would be most beneficial when accompanied by changes in the person's outlook and attitudes that enable him or her more fully to enjoy the activities. See Needles & Abramson (1990).*

in an ever-larger and often fragmented society. You might recall the example of my patient who rather systematically examined the notices of community organizations and joined a hiking club. This is certainly a reasonable approach. In metropolitan areas, there are usually plenty of groups like this to choose from. The recreation department in the suburban community in which I live offers classes in activities ranging from archery to yoga. Churches offer social activities. Some community colleges are becoming meccas for adults seeking to upgrade their skills and pursue their interests. When you get involved in such activities, you increase the opportunities for making new friends.

Research shows that many people who become depressed do not have fluent social skills. They may not present themselves well or feel at ease with other people.[10] The point has to be made that social skills, like most other skills, may improve considerably with practice. Isolating yourself to avoid discomfort and discouragement will not afford you the opportunity to make this improvement.

Some thoughts for people who are feeling depressed: When you meet new friends, projecting gloom and low self-esteem will probably turn people off. You will probably have more success if you can get out of yourself and the problems that have been consuming you and focus your attention on what other people are saying. There is an added benefit to this. One of the surest ways to make new friends is to be a *good listener.*

If you project the feeling that you are really interested in what the other person is saying, you will find yourself in increasing demand. Think of each person that you meet as a special individual who has a unique story to tell, with experiences and ideas that might be interesting to learn about. If you follow this advice, you might be tempted to ask people a ton of questions. This really isn't necessary. A few general questions are usually enough. And one thing to avoid are pointed questions. Such questions can make people defensive.

At a party, a man asked a woman who taught at a high school experiencing some bad problems, "Isn't it awful working there?" The woman became uncomfortable and soon broke off the conversation. The man might have phrased the question, "How do you like working there?" Chances are the conversation would have continued.

In projecting an attitude that you are interested in what the other per-

[10]*See for example Libet & Lewinsohn (1973).*

son is saying, you will probably find it helpful to maintain some eye contact, to nod your head occasionally to indicate that you are paying attention, and – perhaps most importantly – to remember what the other person is saying so that your comments and reactions reflect this. Referring to names, places and ideas that a person has brought up tells the person that you are really tuned in.

It's easier to make and keep friends if one maintains a latitude of tolerance both towards others and oneself. If you look at almost any individual through a microscope, you can usually find something that is "wrong." As we indicated earlier, perfectionism in the choice of friends is about as useful as perfectionist demands on oneself. One may end up without friends.

The starting point in making friends is the attitude that people are different, most people are interesting and good social relationships can enrich your life. Can some people be irritating and a pain in the neck? You bet! But the alternative to trying to develop lasting friendships is isolation, loneliness and increased risk of depression.

A Passing Suggestion

In talking about friendship and attachment, I would like to pass on the idea that the antidepressant buffering effects of having someone around can extend to the companionship of animals. The importance of pets in the lives of many people is a commonplace observation. For people who are fond of animals, pets can have therapeutic value.

In discussing the inclusion of animals in therapeutic programs, Jeff Meer noted that the practice is already in wide use with learning disabled and physically disabled people. Horseback riding is now an adjunct to therapy with these groups in many areas of the country. In Florida, dolphins have been used to encourage communication with autistic children. Meer mentions research carried out by Samuel and Elizabeth Corson.[11] The Corsons used dogs with patients who had not responded to psychotherapy for depression. Almost all of the patients improved after contact with the animals.

If you enjoy animals and are willing to take the time and effort to care for them, you might want to consider this option.

[11]*Described in Meer's (1984) article, p. 62.*

Maintaining a Good Balance in Your Life

We have discussed adding more pleasant experiences in your life and increasing your social activities. These steps are likely to have an antidepressant effect. Implicit in this advice is the notion that all of us have a kind of optimal balance point in our lives—a balance between our various needs—whether the needs be for love and affection, for being with friends, for creative activities, to work on a job, to spend time with children, to exercise, or to spend quiet time alone or in religious observances. Each person's balance of activities is different, depending on how strong one's needs are in different areas. Regardless of the nature of our activities, it is important to try to maintain our different activities at levels that keep us reasonably close to our ideal balance.

Putting all one's eggs into a single basket and letting everything else go is a recipe for emotional distress for many people. If you live for your work or for that passionate love affair, you are putting yourself at risk if something goes wrong. Ask yourself, "If things go badly, what will you have left?" If you take some pains to keep a balance of meaningful activities in your life, you should have a cushion if disappointments happen in one area of your life, a cushion that will help sustain you while you try to fix the things that have gone wrong.

Maintaining a balance in activities helps keep good things happening in life and guards against developing a victim or martyr mentality, which may happen when one is consumed by a single, overriding role in life. When there is more in your life to experience, the chances of experiencing overwhelming disappointment and depression are less. So, set a proper balance for your activities and try not to get too far away from it. If you find yourself becoming too one-sided in your behavior, take steps to bring yourself back to the balance of activities that works best for you.

To briefly recapitulate, the self-help plan I have outlined consists of a number of interrelated ideas. These ideas include (1) setting reasonable but satisfying goals, (2) analyzing the pattern of your daily activities to identify sources of satisfaction and stress-provoking situations, (3) recognizing maladaptive thought patterns which promote problems, and changing these to patterns that promote more positive emotional health, (4) making changes in your life to increase your level of satisfaction, and (5) creating a more optimal balance among your daily activities.

The types of actions I propose are drawn from research and clinical experience and are not unique to this writer. Similar ideas for ways of better handling the pressures of daily life have been advanced by other writers. For example, a recent article by Donald Jewell and Maureen Mylander is very much along these lines.

What I am suggesting represents movement toward a more problem-solving approach to life. Remember that people who become depressed often react in dysfunctional ways, such as catastrophizing situations. These dysfunctional responses can be steps on the path to depression. A path away from depression requires a different approach, beginning with a careful analysis of what has gotten you into trouble and then taking steps to move in new and more constructive directions.

Dr. Arthur Nezu and his colleagues have been using a problem-solving approach in successfully treating depressed patients. They believe, as I do, that it is important to help depressed individuals identify the situations that are causing, or have caused, stress in their lives and to increase the patient's effectiveness in coping with these situations. They have developed a very interesting program that teaches problem-solving skills to patients to help them deal more effectively with future problems.[12]

Along somewhat different lines, researchers have been working on the development of self-help manuals for people who are depressed. Some of these manuals have proven useful in preliminary studies. While not all of these materials are widely available, there are some publications that you might find interesting to examine. An example is a book by Peter Lewinsohn and his colleagues, entitled *Control Your Depression*, which presents a behavioral approach to depression.

James Mahalik and Dennis Kivlighan raised the interesting question of what sorts of persons are likely to profit from using self-help manuals for depression. They carried out a study on mildly depressed students using a self-help manual that laid out a seven-week therapeutic program. The researchers also gave the students personality tests. The investigators found that persons who were "realistic types" seemed to benefit more from the program. The researchers also suggested that persons "who persevere in situations that are challenging and require effort succeed in self-help programs that ask its user to go it alone."[13]

---

[12]*Nezu's approach is described in a number of articles as well as a book. See Nezu et al. (1989), and Nezu et al (1990).*
[13]*Mahalik & Kivlighan (1988), p. 241.*

Obviously, going it alone is not for everyone. But there is really no reason you have to go it alone. While the suggestions advanced in this chapter were offered in the context of self-help, they may also be implemented with the assistance of friends and family or serve as a supplement to psychotherapy. The idea that one does not have to go it alone has become institutionalized in our society in the form of support groups for various disorders. You can find support groups for problems ranging from diabetes to addictions. You will also find groups in many communities that offer support for persons who are depressed. Many of these groups are part of a national organization called the National Depressive and Manic Depressive Association, whose current address is Merchandise Mart, Box 3395, Chicago, IL 60654. Local chapters of this organization offer such things as basic information about the depressive disorders in introductory groups, meetings where members can discuss issues related to the illness, and groups for family members in which they can explore their own feelings about the problem. If you are interested in finding out whether there is a similar society in your area, you might try contacting your local health department or the national society in Chicago.

BIBLIOGRAPHY

Allgood-Merten, B.; Lewinsohn, P. M.; & Hops, H. (1990). Sex differences and adolescent depression. *Journal of Abnormal Psychology, 99,* 55–63.

Berscheid, E.; Walster, E.; & Bohrnstedt, G. (1973, November). The happy American body: A survey report. *Psychology Today, 7,* 119–31.

Cash, T. F.; Winstead, B. A.; & Janda, L. H. (1986, April). The great American shape-up. *Psychology Today, 20,* 30–37.

Christensen, L., & Burrows, R. (1990). Dietary treatment of depression. *Behavior Therapy, 21,* 183–93.

Hewitt, P. L., & Flett, G. L. (1991). Dimensions of perfectionism in unipolar depression. *Journal of Abnormal Psychology, 100,* 98–101.

Jewell, D. S., & Mylander, M. (1988). The psychology of stress: Run silent, run deep. In G. P. Chorousos, D. L. Loriaux, and P. W. Gold (eds.), *Mechanisms of Physical and Emotional Stress.* New York: Plenum.

Keats, J. (1958). *The poetical works of John Keats.* Oxford: Oxford University Press.

Lewinsohn, P. M.; Munoz, R. F.; Youngren, M. A.; & Zeiss, A. M. (1986). *Control your depression.* Englewood Cliffs, N.J.: Prentice Hall.

Libet, J. M., & Lewinsohn, P. M. (19873). The concept of social skills with special reference to the behavior of depressed persons. *Journal of Consulting and Clinical Psychology,* 40, 304–12.

Mahalik, J. R., & Kivlighan, D. M., Jr. (1988). Self-help treatment for depression: Who succeeds? *Journal of Counseling Psychology,* 35, 237–42.

Meer, J. (1984, August). Pet theories. *Psychology Today,* 18, 60–67.

National Depressive and Manic-Depressive Association Newsletter. (1989, winter).

Needles, D. J., & Abramson, L. Y. (1990). Positive life events, attributional style, and hopefulness: Testing a model of recovery from depression. *Journal of Abnormal Psychology,* 99, 156–65.

Nezu, A. M.; Nezu, C. M.; & Perri, M. G. (1989). *Problem-solving therapy for depression: Theory, research and clinical guidelines.* New York: Wiley.

_____; _____; & _____ (1990). Psychotherapy for adults within a problem-solving framework: Focus on depression. *Journal of Cognitive Psychotherapy,* 4, 247–56.

Noles, S. W.; Cash, T. F.; & Winstead, B. A. (1985). Body image, physical attractiveness, and depression. *Journal of Consulting and Clinical Psychology,* 53, 88–94.

Simons, A. D.; Epstein, L. H.; McGowan, C. R.; & Kuper, D. J. (1985). Exercise as a treatment for depression: An update. *Clinical Psychology Review,* 5, 533–68.

Solomon, M. R. (1986, April). Dress for effect. *Psychology Today,* 20, 20–28.

Spring, B.; Chiodo, J.; & Bowen, D. J. (1987). Carbohydrates, tryptophan, and behavior: A methodological review. *Psychological Bulletin,* 102, 234–56.

Veleber, D. M., & Templer, D. I. (1984). Effects of caffeine on anxiety and depression. *Journal of Abnormal Psychology,* 93, 120–22.

Weick, K. E. (1984). Small wins: Redefining the scale of social problems. *American Psychologist,* 39, 40–49.

9. Some Counsel for the Family and Friends of a Depressed Person

In earlier chapters, I discussed how family and friends can be the sources of stress that trigger a depressive reaction. Paradoxically, we also saw how family and friends can be a buffer, shielding a vulnerable person from experiencing a depressive reaction. Let's see if we can unravel this seeming contradiction.

Difficulties in interpersonal relationships are among the more significant stressors that we encounter. These stresses may arise in a parent-child relationship where the child suffers at the hands of an unaffectionate, neglectful or abusive parent. Sometimes, the shoe may be on the other foot. Consider the stresses generated in parents whose teenage children become involved in drugs or delinquency. The stresses of romantic love with its passions, disappointments and breakups sometimes are overwhelming. The stresses of a bad marriage can lead to an emotional debacle for both parties.

When relationships are destructive, they are part of the problem in depression. When they are not, they are part of the solution. Fortunately, most of us have relationships that have a lot of good in them. We are not talking about perfect relationships; we are talking about relationships where there are *positive bonds,* and whatever difficulties exist are manageable. Perhaps the critical factors are a *feeling of belongingness* – a feeling that these are my people – and a *sense of support* – a sense of assurance that they are here for me in times of trouble.

The concept of bonds is basic to human security. Remember the attachment that infants develop as a basis for beginning their exploration of the unknown environment about them. The need to be related to others remains with us in varying degrees for the rest of our days. People who have close, positive relationships tend to be happier and healthier. Married people are more likely to live longer than single people. If good relationships are a prophylaxis for depression, the question becomes "How can we best utilize such relationships to assist those who are vulnerable to depressive problems?" Or put very simply, "How can family members or good friends help?"

The first key to being helpful is to understand. Understanding begins with being knowledgeable about depression. Here is a brief checklist of some important things to keep in mind about depression.

1. Remember the symptoms of depression. Understand the difference between transitory depressed mood and depressive disorder. If depressed symptoms *persist*, there is a problem that needs attention.
2. Remember that there are different types of depression. While most depressions are unipolar, some people have bipolar disorder. The symptoms of bipolar disorder are different and the treatment is different.
3. Keep in mind that depression often has a genetic basis. Some people have inherited vulnerabilities and are more likely to react with depression than others. Remember that the mechanisms for depression are in part biological, including disturbances in the action of the neurotransmitters in the brain.
4. Remember that stressors often trigger depression.
5. Keep in mind that support from friends and loved ones is very good medicine for depression.

Knowledge about depression is most useful when it is translated into *alertness* that there is a problem in your family and friends and that something needs to be done. When you recognize clear signs of depression in persons close to you, it may prove helpful if you can find out what mental health resources are available in your community so you can offer reasoned advice when the opportunity seems appropriate. Find out about the availability of psychiatrists, psychologists, clinical social workers and mental health support groups.

When things are clearly going wrong, you can suggest going for a professional consultation, perhaps starting with the family doctor. If the troubled person feels unsure, consider volunteering to go along with the person. The important thing is that you do whatever you can *reasonably* do to ensure that the person who needs help gets it.

If you make a suggestion that someone should consult a professional for a depressive problem, you may well run into resistance. You may hear responses like, "I don't need help," or "Nobody can help me, there's nothing anyone can do." These statements may reflect the confusion, hopelessness and inertia that are part of the depressive problem.

One approach to dealing with such resistance is to first make it clear that you recognize the pain and suffering that the person is going through and what a difficult problem it is. Try to communicate the idea that "I understand that you're going through a lot of pain and I want to help." Then you might state that there are a variety of treatments available that are effective for most people who have depressive problems. Explain that there are different kinds of medicine and short-term psychotherapies that have proven useful. One of these treatments may help him or her feel better.

Alertness on your part as a member of the family or close friend should extend beyond recognizing the need for outside help and suggesting that the person seek it. When a person is severely depressed, alertness also means keeping an eye open for potential signs of self-inflicted harm. The possibility of suicide is a very troubling idea, but you must be aware of it. While no one can predict with any certainty when a seriously depressed person might make a suicidal attempt, there are a number of signs that suggest the possibility of one. Here are three signs that are particularly worrisome.

1. The person expresses feelings of hopelessness. He or she sees the future as bleak and sees "no way out."
2. The person talks openly about suicide. There may be statements like "I can't stand this pain anymore" or "I won't be around."
3. The person has made a previous suicide attempt.

The first sign suggests a state of thorough demoralization. Charles Neuringer painted a portrait of such demoralization in describing a group of women who threatened suicide after experiencing a personal crisis.

> They felt life to be duller, emptier, and more boring than the other women did. They also seemed less interested and responsive to people and to events than did the other groups. They felt angrier than the other participants; they had less interest in their work and were more dissatisfied with it than were the other women. Their thought processes were experienced as slow and sluggish,

which was not true for the other participants. They felt that thinking was a great effort and that their ideas were valueless. . . . The high-lethality women felt more anxious than the others. They also felt more guilt-ridden and were less self-approving than the other women. Their feelings of inadequacy and helplessness were greater than those of the other participants. They also felt more depressed and weary than the other women.[1]

No matter how careful family and friends try to be, there is always a chance of self-inflicted tragedy. A survey of psychologists revealed that about one-quarter of them had a patient who committed suicide while under their care. The emotional effects of this tragedy on the psychologists were severe. The effects on members of the family can be devastating.

As a general rule, it seems unfair to hold anyone responsible for another person's suicide. A therapist may see a patient for an hour or two a week. Members of the family have a multitude of other responsibilities. It is virtually impossible to prevent a suicide by someone who is determined to carry out the act, unless the person is hospitalized and kept under 24-hour surveillance. The crucial thing would be to know when to hospitalize, and we simply do not have the scientific basis to allow us to know this with certainty.

If a patient exhibits signs of suicide, then family consultation with the attending physician and or therapist seems warranted. A decision by the patient and the therapist for *voluntary hospitalization* may be in order. Hospitalization would last until the crisis is over and the high risk of suicide has abated.

If there is a high risk of suicide and the patient is unwilling to be hospitalized, a very difficult situation emerges. The options are to live with a high risk or to set into motion the coercive power of the state to hospitalize the patient against his or her will. This can be a very unpleasant dilemma; it is not only a wrenching emotional experience but places one in a briar patch of ethical and legal thorns.

Maverick psychiatrist Thomas Szasz has suggested that it is questionable for mental health professionals to get into the business of suicide prevention, suggesting that "forcibly imposed interventions to prevent suicide deprive the patient of liberty and dignity" and that "the use of psychiatric coercion to prevent suicide is at once impractical and immoral."[2]

[1]*Neuringer (1982), p. 185.*
[2]*Szasz (1986), p. 809.*

I think one has to recognize that the thought of suicide in depressed people comes near the bottom of a psychological well, probably exacerbated by biological dysregulation. It is not a condition in which one expects to find rational decision making. A few weeks of time and treatment may make the world look very different to the patient. The argument for intervention is to allow this change of attitude to happen.

Learning about depression and community mental health resources, and becoming alert to signs of depression in those who are close to you are constructive steps to take in being of help to loved ones or friends who are experiencing a depressive problem. Recognition of strains and stressors in the home environment is another important area where family members may be particularly helpful. Try to become aware of any environmental problems and interpersonal strains that are exacerbating the stress levels of the patient. If there are chronic hassles in the home situation that are irritating the patient, can something be done to defuse them? Stress-free environments are not reasonable goals, but lowering levels of stress certainly are. If a member of the family is doing something roughly equivalent to beating on a drum all day long, maybe you can do something to stop it. A more peaceful environment may be a good idea for everyone.

It may be a time to look inward, too. Is there anything you might be doing that is exacerbating the problem, something that is causing stress for the patient. Give it some thought. If there is, would it be possible to make some changes?

As a person who is concerned about depression in a friend or loved one, you might have as one of your objectives to increase your *sensitivity* to the concerns, thinking processes and feelings of the person. What this comes down to in large part is better listening, paying attention to what is said and trying to put yourself into the shoes of the other person so you can better understand what is happening. When you do this, the other person will sense that you care and you will have increased understanding of the problem.

If the depressed person is undergoing psychotherapy, the spouse may be asked to come in for one or more sessions. Many therapists like to do this, as it enables them to see the patient's behavior from another perspective. As family problems and particularly marital conflicts can play a role in triggering depressive episodes, it sometimes makes good sense to try to deal with these problems as part of therapy. If these difficulties cannot be resolved to a reasonable degree, the chances are high that there will be further episodes of depression in the future. Interestingly, marital therapy itself, in which the focus is on both parties, can sometimes be as effective in treating depression as therapy focused on the depressed person.[3]

If it becomes clear in therapy that changes are needed in the patient's life-style, there may be an opportunity for you to participate in making these changes. For example, exercise usually has antidepressive effects. How about starting a walking or jogging program or some other exercise program on a regular basis with the patient? As we have emphasized, it should be exercise that is approved by the family physician and something you both enjoy.

There may be a need to introduce more pleasant activities into the patient's life. You can help in arranging that dinner out, that ride in the countryside, that visit with friends or whatever the two of you feel is fun and not too stressful. These activities should be paced into the recovery process as part of a plan to establish a more balanced life-style.

As you do these things, it is important to recognize signs of resistance and not to push too hard when you detect them. Go with what works and build on successes. A little praise on your part when there has been progress may help keep things moving along.

The behavior of depressed persons turns off many people; the sad expression, the tears, the stream of self-deprecatory comment, the pessimism and hopelessness can be difficult to take. There will be times when you may be tempted to throw in the towel and give up trying to help. Try not to do that. Remember, most people who are depressed usually get better. Some people get better even without medication or therapy. Moreover, drugs and psychotherapy are both proven means of helping patients overcome episodes of depression. It is important to keep in mind that even when things look bleakest, the odds for most people are that the symptoms will abate and the afflicted individual will become a good deal better.

While not giving up is the marching order of the day, the spouse and children of a depressed person may have to take steps to protect their own mental health during the depressive episode. Living with a person who is depressed can be very difficult. If the illness is a protracted one, the task can wear down the spouse, family members and friends. The spouse and children run a risk of developing emotional problems of their

[3]See Beach (1987).

own. In carrying out research on persons living with depressed individuals, James Coyne and his colleagues observed, "Overall, 40% of the respondents living with a depressed person in the midst of an episode were sufficiently distressed themselves to meet the criterion for needing psychological intervention."[4] With this magnitude of risk, it is prudent for the spouse and children to do things to protect themselves from being overwhelmed by the problem.

Some obvious suggestions are getting away from the house at times, doing things that the individuals enjoy. Perhaps it is spending time with friends, going for a walk, or taking in a movie. The objectives are to keep one's own routines as normal as possible during the illness and to divert oneself from the problem to keep it from reaching overwhelming proportions. You can't help the distressed member of the family if you are going under yourself. Caretakers need a safety valve too: few people are emotionally indestructible.

If there are young children in the family, the intact spouse has the responsibility of insulating them from the more emotionally destructive effects of the illness. It is not going to do the children any good to spend a lot of time with a parent in the depths of a depressive episode. Try to find things for the children to do when things are bad. Look for means of getting them out of harm's way. When the situation improves, the children can be helpful in the recovery.

BIBLIOGRAPHY

Beach, S. R. H.; Sandeen, E. E.; & O'Leary, K. D. (1987, November). Treatment for the depressed maritally discordant client: A comparison of behavioral marital therapy, individual cognitive thrapy, and wait list. Paper presented at the annual meeting of the Association for the Advancement of Behavior Therapy, Boston, Massachusetts.

Beck, A. T.; Brown, G.; & Steer, R. A. (1989). Prediction of eventual suicide in psychiatric inpatients by clinical ratings of hopelessness. *Journal of Consulting and Clinical Psychology, 57*, 309–10.

Coyne, J. C.; Kessler, R. C.; Tal, M.; Turnbull, J.; Wortman, C. B.; & Greden, J. F. (1987). Living with a depressed person. *Journal of Consulting and Clinical Psychology, 55*, 347–52.

Howes, M. J., & Hokanson, J. E. (1979). Conversational and social responses to

[4]*Coyne et al. (1987), p. 350.*

depressive interpersonal behavior. *Journal of Abnormal Psychology,* 88, 625–34.

Neuringer, C. (1982). Affect configurations and changes in women who threaten suicide following a crisis. *Journal of Consulting and Clinical Psychology,* 50, 182–86.

Shneidman, E. (1987, March). At the point of no return. *Psychology Today,* 21, 54–58.

Szasz, T. (1986). The case against suicide prevention. *American Psychologist,* 41, 806–12.

10. Professional Help

When Erica's husband, Jack, began having problems, Erica didn't know what to make of them. Jack had trouble falling asleep at night. When Erica awoke at night, she saw him lying there wide awake. Sometimes he would get up and pace the floor. In the morning there were circles under his eyes; he looked exhausted. Jack used to be a big eater, but now his appetite had dwindled. Breakfast was no more than coffee and it seemed that he hardly touched his dinner. Jack looked sad and at times he brooded. He complained of headaches and stomach cramps. He said he had no energy to do anything and worse, he didn't seem interested in doing anything. They used to go bowling every Friday night and visit her mother on Sunday. Now he didn't want to do either. And his interest in her sexually had almost disappeared.

Erica knew something was wrong, but didn't know what it was or what to do about it. She confided in her sister Robin, who suggested that Jack see the doctor. When Erica broached the idea to Jack, he resisted it, but she kept at it and finally Jack consulted his physician, Dr. Sutherland. Dr. Sutherland was in the midst of a very busy day. He listened to Jack for a few minutes and thought Jack sounded like a "croc," a patient with lots of complaints without any physical basis for them. Dr. Sutherland ordered some routine lab tests. When all tests proved negative, he suggested that Jack take a few days off from work and see if he felt better. In his brief examination, Dr. Sutherland did not identify the problem for what it was: depression.

We might recall the study carried out in the VA hospital on elderly patients where only 2 of 23 depressed patients were correctly identified by the house staff as being depressed.[1] As physicians are often the gatekeepers for people needing professional help in the treatment of

[1]*Rapp et al. (1988).*

145

emotional problems, it is obviously important that physicians be able to recognize such problems and recommend appropriate treatment. Noting the role that family physicians can play in treatment and referral, the National Institute of Mental Health is stepping up its efforts in physician education concerning depression.

Jack's short vacation helped only a little. When he began to have difficulties on his job and wanted more time off, Jack spoke to the counselor in the personnel office at work. She talked with Jack several times, then recommended that he consult a therapist. She gave him the names of a psychiatrist and a psychologist who had worked with other employees in the company who had emotional problems. Jack was able to get an early appointment with the psychologist. When Jack began therapy he became one of some ten million people who made a visit that year for professional mental health care.

Despite these numbers, getting the kind of help needed for treatment of mental and emotional disorders is not as straightforward a task as it might seem. If Jack's symptoms had been bizarre, such as the delusions that occur in schizophrenia, or if he had behaved violently, his family and friends might have more easily recognized that he needed the care of mental health professionals. But depression is not that easy to identify.

As it turned out, Jack and Erica were fortunate because the counselor at Jack's place of employment was able to steer him to a mental health practitioner. For many people, the road to getting help is rockier, with more than one misstep.

It may be a friend, a family member, a clergyman or the family physician who eventually provides the needed guidance. It may come down to a friend who says something like "I had a bad problem, myself. I saw Dr. Johnson. She helped me a lot. I'll give you her number. Maybe she can help you, too."

Researchers have found that the great majority of people with emotional problems discuss their problems with friends or relatives before seeking professional help from a mental health practitioner.[2] What seems to make a difference in influencing the troubled person to seek professional help is whether the friend or relative has some knowledge of, or experience with, the mental health profession. If a friend mentions counseling, the distressed person is more likely to seek it.

[2]*See Yokopenic et al. (1983).*

Mental Health Services in the United States

Let's take a look at the availability of mental health services in the United States. In 1980, close to ten million persons made one or more visits to a professional for mental health care.[3] About half of these consultations were visits to the office of a psychiatrist or psychologist. Many people also went to organized care settings such as community mental health clinics or outpatient care departments of hospitals.

The numbers of people visiting mental health professionals may seem large, but it is not the whole story by any means. Many people who need professional mental health care simply don't get it. It has been estimated that about 15 percent of the population needs mental health treatment.[4] Perhaps a fifth of these people — and that means many millions — do not see any professionals either in the health care or mental health care systems for their problems. About half of the people with emotional disorders do see a doctor, but do not see anyone with specialized mental health training. Only about one out of five persons with a mental or emotional disorder enter treatment with a mental health professional. In regard to depression, one survey indicated that most people suffering from depression do not seek professional help.[5] Under-utilization is particularly noticeable among minority groups. For example, a survey found that Mexican American persons with a diagnosed mental disorder were only half as likely to see a mental health professional as non–Hispanic Whites.[6] The reasons for the gap between need and help received include the public's lack of information about depression, the cost of mental health services, and their availability.

Therapy for depression is expensive. Visits to psychiatrists, psychologists and clinical social workers may run $50, $60, $70, $80 or even more. The cost, however, may appear more excessive at first than it is. Many health insurance plans cover depression and will pay a substantial part of the cost. Short-term therapies running over a few months are usually effective for depression. Lower cost help may also be available in community mental health centers.

If you are looking for a professionally trained person to help you with

[3]See Taube et al. (1984), p. 1437.
[4]See Regier et al. (1978) for a discussion of statistics relating to the need for and utilization of mental health services.
[5]See Weissman et al. (1981).
[6]See Hough et al. (1987).

your depression problem, you will have a much greater chance of finding a qualified person in some areas of the United States than in others. If you live in an urban area that has substantial resources you should have little difficulty finding help. Psychiatrists, psychologists and clinical social workers congregate in urban areas where people are better educated, earn higher incomes and have health insurance that can help pay for the cost of therapy. There are plenty of therapists in urban centers like New York City and Washington, D.C. However, if you happen to live in a smaller, less affluent county, you may not find a single psychiatrist, psychologist or clinical social worker available. A study reported in 1984 indicated that there are more counties in the United States without any mental health providers than there are counties with providers.[7] For persons in rural America, it may be a very long drive for that weekly session with a therapist.

In professional mental health care there are several options for the treatment of depression. These include antidepressive medications, psychotherapy, and inpatient hospitalization. For mild to moderate levels of depression, therapy and or medication are reasonable choices. For a person who is very seriously depressed and is suicidal, hospitalization may be necessary.

Medication for Depression

Antidepressive medications may be prescribed only by a physician. A family physician may do this as well as a psychiatrist. Antidepressive medications are effective for most, but not all, patients. Like most drugs, antidepressant medications may cause side effects. Patients differ in how well they can tolerate antidepressant drugs and some patients are not able to use the drugs.

Antidepressant drugs are now widely used. Surveys indicate that during a recent year about 2 percent of adult Americans took an antidepressant medicine.[8] It is estimated that between 20 and 30 million prescriptions for antidepressants were filled in U.S. pharmacies in a single year. The drugs that have been most often used in treating unipolar

[7]See Knesper et al. (1984).
[8]These estimates based on a NIMH survey are cited in Folkenberg (1983).

depression are called *tricyclics*. Tricyclics have an effect on the neurotransmitter systems, which may be the basis for their positive effects on depression. There are a number of tricyclics in current clinical use. The list includes Amitriptyline, Amoxapine, Desipramine, Imipramine and Trimipramine. Some more familiar trade names for these chemicals include Elavil, Norpramine and Tofranil, to name a few.

You can see that there are a variety of tricyclic medications to choose from. It is possible that if a patient does not respond to one of these antidepressants, another drug could still prove beneficial. It is also possible that if a patient experiences unpleasant side effects from one drug, another drug may prove more acceptable.

As tricyclics can be dangerous in excessive amounts, patients should not unilaterally increase the dose beyond what their doctor has prescribed. Overdoses of tricyclics have been noted in hospital emergency rooms, sometimes as a method of attempted suicide, sometimes out of ignorance of the power of the drugs.[9] A patient might have the mistaken notion that if a small amount of the drug is helpful, a larger amount of the drug would be even more helpful. Some of the side effects of tricyclics that have been reported are weight gain, dizziness, blurred vision, sweating, constipation, sedation and, in some patients, cardiovascular problems.

A panel of experts created by the National Institutes of Health issued some consensus recommendations for the use of antidepressant drugs. For example, the panel recommended that when a decision is made to discontinue the use of tricyclics, the drug should be phased out over a period of time to avoid problems that might occur if the drug is discontinued abruptly. The recommendation was that a large drop in dose level should occur in the early stage of the withdrawal process and then the dosage of the drug should be gradually tapered off.

It may take some time before the benefits of tricyclics can be observed. Tricyclics are believed to be effective in alleviating a number of the symptoms of depression. An NIMH bulletin, *Depressive Disorders: Treatments Bring New Hope*, states, "The tricyclics alleviate such symptoms as loss of appetite and weight, decreased capacity to feel pleasure, loss of energy, psychomotor retardation, suicidal thoughts, and thought patterns dominated by hopelessness, helplessness, and excessive guilt."[10] Tricyclics appear to be useful in helping many patients shake off the

[9]*See Kathol & Henn (1983).*
[10]*Sargent (1986), p. 13.*

lethargy of depression, helping to get patients moving again. These drugs do not solve the interpersonal and environmental problems that may have precipitated the depression. While tricyclics help a majority of depressed patients, they do not help all patients.

The following example of a clinical study demonstrates the beneficial effects of tricyclics on depression. Imipramine hydrochloride, with brand names such as Tofranil, is a frequently used tricyclic antidepressant medication. A research team led by James Kocsis wanted to evaluate the effectiveness of this drug in treating depression. For their study they recruited subjects from among adults who sought outpatient treatment for depression at two medical centers, one in New York, the other in Maine. The subjects were screened by psychiatrists to make sure they met the currently established criteria for chronic unipolar depression and had not been on antidepressant medications during the preceding six months.

All patients who were accepted into the study were given placebo tablets for two weeks. These tablets had the same appearance as the imipramine tablets but had no therapeutic action. At the end of two weeks, the patients were randomly assigned either to continue with the placebo or to receive imipramine. In a "double blind" design, neither the patients nor the evaluating psychiatrists knew who had been given the medication and who had been given the placebo.

After six weeks, the patients were reevaluated. The patients who showed a substantial improvement in their depressive symptoms were called "responders." The patients who did not were called "non-responders." The results: 59 percent of the patients given imipramine and 13 percent of the patients given the placebo were characterized as responders. The study shows that imipramine can be an effective antidepressant with many patients, though clearly not with all.

Another type of antidepressant drug is called *MAO inhibitors.* MAO in this case stands for monoamine oxidase, an enzyme in the body chemistry that breaks down neurotransmitter molecules into inactive substances. It would seem that for many depressed patients it would be beneficial to interfere with this breakdown process and preserve these useful molecules. MAO inhibitors do this. Some chemical names for MAO inhibitors are phenelzine, tranylcypromine and isocarboxazid.

There are some problems in using MAO inhibitors. When patients take MAO inhibitors, it is important for them to watch their diet very carefully, for certain foods could trigger serious cardiovascular problems.

Among the foods on the avoidance list are beer, red wine, chocolate, pickled fish, cheese and yogurt. Patients on MAO inhibitors may also have to avoid caffeine and allergy medicines.

MAO inhibitors are believed to be particularly useful for patients with "atypical depressions"—i.e., depressive problems that don't show some of the usual symptoms of unipolar depression. For example, MAO inhibitors may be beneficial for patients who are overly drowsy and who overeat. MAO inhibitors may also be useful for depressed patients who are experiencing high levels of anxiety or whose symptom patterns include other types of emotional problems such as phobias or obsessive-compulsive behaviors. Researchers studying the effects of MAO inhibitors on patients diagnosed as having atypical depression have reported a number of beneficial effects. MAO inhibitors have done such things as improve the patient's mood, reduce guilt feelings and feelings of helplessness and perk up interest in work and activities. The medication has also lessened feelings of anxiety.[11]

Fluoxetine hydrochloride, better known by the brand name Prozac, is a new, different type of antidepressant drug. In its informational monograph on Prozac, the drug's producer Eli Lilly and Company notes that Prozac is "chemically unrelated and pharmacologically distinct from tricyclic" antidepressants.[12]

Prozac is believed to have the effect of increasing the concentration of the neurotransmitter serotonin in the synaptic portions of the brain. Compared to the tricyclic drugs, fluoxetine hydrochloride acts selectively on the neurotransmitters; its action is relatively specific for the serotonin pathway. The drug has little effect on the uptake of other neurotransmitters. The selectivity of Prozac has advantages in avoiding adverse reactions that may arise from modifying the actions of the other neurotransmitter systems. An antidepressant drug that combines effectiveness with fewer side effects is a very attractive package.

How effective is Prozac? The studies cited in the Lilly monograph indicate that the drug is comparable in effectiveness to some of the tricyclic drugs (e.g., imipramine) in reducing symptoms of depression. As far as side effects go, Lilly reports a lower incidence of reactions associated with tricyclics, such as cardiac effects, dry mouth, drowsiness, dizziness, and weight gain.

[11]*See Davidson et al. (1988).*
[12]*Prozac (1990).*

With this performance in clinical trials, Prozac has become a widely prescribed drug in a very short time. Press reports estimate that sales are in the range of a million prescriptions a month. The drug has been featured in a cover story in *Newsweek*.[13] A few words of caution, however, should be thrown in. Lilly points out that little is known about the long-term efficacy of the drug. The use of the drug over periods of months and years has not been fully evaluated.[14] And while Prozac may have fewer of certain side effects than tricyclics, the drug is not free from adverse reactions. Significant numbers of users experience such problems as headaches, nausea, insomnia and nervousness.[15] The recommended dose of Prozac is 20 mg per day, though a physician may prescribe higher doses if no improvement is observed. Lilly notes that it may take several weeks for the full therapeutic effect of the drug to be apparent.

The tricyclics, MAO inhibitors and fluoxetine hydrochloride, thus, are medicines that are frequently used in the treatment of unipolar depression. For the treatment of bipolar depression, *lithium* is a drug that has been used extensively. Lithium is a popular name for the chemicals *lithium carbonate* and *lithium citrate*. Lithium compounds are found in some rocks, in the sea and in sparse quantities in the tissues of plants and animals. As a drug, lithium carbonate is taken orally in the form of a capsule or tablet. Some trade names for the drug are Eskalith, Lithane and Lithonate.

An Australian physician, John Cade, used lithium successfully as a treatment for mania in the late 1940s, but his work was not fully exploited until many years later. A major problem with lithium was that if the drug were used at too high a dose, it could have very dangerous effects. When the problems relating to drug safety were resolved, the drug was approved by the FDA for psychiatric use and is now in widespread use.

Lithium is presently considered to be the drug of choice in the treatment of bipolar depression. Lithium has the effect of reducing bipolar mood swings. Something like 3 out of 4 patients with bipolar disorder improve when using lithium.[16] Many patients will stop having manic-

[13]Newsweek, *March 26, 1990, has a lengthy article on Prozac.*

[14]*Longer range studies are in process. Personal communication, Eli Lilly and Company.*

[15]*See Prozac (1990), pp. 17–23. One other possible caution about the drug was voiced in a report that noted a preoccupation with suicide among six depressed patients using the drug. See Teicher (1990). Newer antidepressant drugs also include trazodone and bupropion.*

[16]*See Sargent (1986), p. 14.*

depressive episodes. In other patients, the episodes will be fewer in number, shorter in length or less severe. Because lithium is toxic at high dosage levels, the dose for the individual patient must be carefully determined. It has to be high enough to be therapeutic, but below the range of toxicity.

In clinical practice, the patient's physician will take blood tests periodically to monitor the amount of lithium in the blood. Because this level increases rapidly during the first few hours after the drug is taken, blood tests must be delayed for a number of hours before an accurate measure can be ascertained. In carrying out these tests, a patient will usually take lithium at night and have blood drawn at the doctor's office in the morning.

Lithium may have a number of unpleasant side effects. Upon beginning lithium therapy, some patients report such problems as nausea, stomach cramps, thirst, muscle weakness and tiredness. Some patients develop a tremor in the hand. For many patients, these symptoms may subside after the drug is used for a while. Other side effects of the drug include weight gain and increased urination. Lithium is usually not prescribed for patients with kidney problems or patients using diuretics. It is important for patients using lithium to work closely with their physician when they begin using the drug and to follow the physician's instructions carefully in the continued use of the drug.

In addition to the physiological side effects listed, lithium can have some effect on both motor speed and memory. In one study, patients on lithium were given a test of motor speed—tapping a telegraphlike key. When the patients were taken off the drug, they performed the task quicker; lithium seemed to slow the patients' performance.[17] The patients' ability to recall an experimental list of words was also poorer while they were using the drug. Lithium did not affect immediate recall of the words, but had an effect on recall for the words when the patients were tested at a later date.[18] For many people, a modest drop in motor performance or long-term memory might have little significance in their daily lives. However, one can imagine that in certain jobs that require hand speed, lithium use could conceivably pose a problem.

Because of the side effects of lithium—or for reasons such as patients feeling they don't need the drug anymore—a great many patients, perhaps

[17]*See Shaw et al. (1987).*
[18]*See Shaw et al. (1987).*

as many as half of those trying the drug, have discontinued its use.[19] For this reason, researchers have been looking for alternative drugs for people who do not respond to lithium or cannot tolerate it.[20] One such medication is an anticonvulsant drug, carbamazepine, which has the brand name Tegretol. The drug appears to be useful for many patients with bipolar depression. Some drugs that have been used in the treatment of hypertension have also received some experimental trials for bipolar depression. It should be stated that none of these drugs are without possible side effects.

Both research and clinical experience lead to the conclusion that antidepressant drugs are important weapons in the treatment of depression for adults. One may wonder whether these drugs may also be useful in the treatment of children who are diagnosed as depressed. The question is not an academic one, for children are being given such drugs in hospitals today.

The treatment for children who are depressed is an unsettled issue. One line of thought is not to overtreat children on the theory that one may be witnessing developmental difficulties that could disappear in time. Some credence for keeping intervention minimal is the good response many depressed children have had to placebos while serving as control subjects in the studies of the effectiveness of antidepressant drugs. The admonition "to do no harm" when treating depression in children should be kept in mind.

Talking and behavioral therapies seem on an intuitive level as the first line of intervention in the treatment of depression in children. Increasing the child's self-esteem and helping the child relate better to other children would be important therapeutic objectives. Pets may be very useful in rebuilding and nurturing the child's capability of forming attachments.

If psychological and behavioral interventions are ineffective, drug therapy is an option to consider. Of the antidepressive drugs, the tricyclics have been used most extensively with children. Evaluation studies indicate that these drugs are usually effective with children, especially when certain plasma levels are achieved in blood tests.[21] The drugs

[19]See Jamison et al. (1979) and Jamison and Akiskal (1983) for discussions of patient compliance with lithium.

[20]For a review of research on carbamazepine and other drug alternatives to lithium in the treatment of bipolar disorder see Prien & Gelenberg (1989).

[21]See Rancurello (1986), p. 179.

seem particularly useful in elevating depressed mood. In reviewing the use of tricyclic antidepressants with children, Michael Rancurello cautions that because of the possibilities of cardiovascular effects from these drugs, electrocardiograms (EKGs) should be taken before and during treatment.

There are some reports indicating that lithium can be used successfully with children who have bipolar depression. However, Rancurello points out that the risk of long-term lithium use are largely unknown, particularly for children who are undergoing rapid growth. Consequently, it seems prudent to reserve the use of the drug until other treatments are shown to be ineffective. With the possible negative effects of antidepressant drugs, there is a compelling need to push foward the development of psychosocial treatments for depression in children and evaluate their effectiveness.

Psychotherapy

Antidepressant drugs have proved helpful for many people in dealing with depressive problems. However, for some of these people, the side effects of the drugs are quite uncomfortable. Moreover, there are many people who are not helped appreciably by these drugs. Fortunately, there is an alternative approach to the treatment of depression, which is drug free. This approach is psychotherapy.

The evidence to date suggests that psychotherapy is as effective a treatment for unipolar depression as medication, and perhaps more so. In reviewing the results of 56 studies, some of which used psychotherapy and some medication, Susan Steinbrueck and her colleagues concluded, "The present findings suggest that in the area of treatment of unipolar depression with adults, psychotherapy appears to be somewhat more effective than drug therapy."[22]

[22]*Steinbrueck, et al. (1983). While this review is clearly encouraging for persons who choose psychotherapy to treat depression, it should be stated that the relative effectiveness of medications and psychotherapy in the treatment of depression is still an unsettled question. For example, in a 1989 review of studies comparing antidepressant drugs with cognitive therapy, Keith Dobson stated that "it appears to be a reliable conclusion that, as assessed by changes in the [Beck Depression Inventory] cognitive therapy is more effective than nothing at all, behavior therapy, or pharmacotherapy in the treatment of clinical depression." Dobson (1989), p. 417. However, a major collaborative investigation carried out under the sponsorship of The National Institute of Mental Health reported* (cont.)

Drugs act on body chemistry to achieve their effects. A drug may have the effect of stabilizing mood swings, as is the case for lithium, or have activating effects on mood and behavior, as is the case for the tricyclics. Psychotherapy has its impact on thoughts, feelings and behavior. Psychotherapy can have significant effects on a person's attitudes and life-style, helping him or her better cope with the interpersonal and environmental stressors that tend to trigger depression.

The question may be raised, "Can drugs and psychotherapy be used together in the treatment of a patient?" The answer is yes. It is a common practice, and research suggests that the combination of these two treatments may be somewhat more effective than either treatment used alone.[23]

While almost all of us are familiar with medicines, many people have only a vague idea of what psychotherapy is. One's image of therapy may be something like the cartoon character of a bearded analyst holding a small notebook, sitting behind a patient who is reclining on a couch, listening to the patient talk at length about what is on his or her mind. While this picture may once have been close to the mark, it is not typical today.

The poet Elizabeth Barrett Browning wrote a memorable sonnet that began, "How do I love thee? Let me count the ways." If she had counted as many ways as there are ways of doing psychotherapy today, her brief sonnet would have turned into a multipaged epic.

A few decades ago the choice in psychotherapy consisted of not much more than several varieties of psychoanalysis and client-centered therapy developed by Carl Rogers. How the situation has changed! Let me quote from an article by Alan Kazdin: "Although at any given time it is difficult to pinpoint the precise number of techniques in use, surveys

(cont. from p. 155) *that a standard reference treatment, the antidepressant drug imipramine plus clinical management was as effective as two forms of psychotherapy—interpersonal therapy and cognitive therapy. See Elkin (1989).*

Some investigators have also raised questions about the adequacy of the research designs that have been used in these comparative studies. In a critique, Steven Hollon and his colleagues (1991) stated, "Nonetheless, questions concerning the representativeness of the samples studied and the adequacy with which pharmacotherapy has been implemented undermine the certainty with which any such conclusions can be drawn." Having said that, they still observed that "with the exception of the recent NIMH collaborative trial, cognitive therapy has performed at least as well as antidepressant pharmacotherapy in virtually every respect in every major comparison."

[23]*See Conte et al. (1986).*

have revealed tremendous growth. In the early 1960s, approximately 60 different types of psychotherapy were identified.... By the mid–1970s, more than 130 techniques were delineated.... By the late 1970s, growth continued to encompass more than 250 techniques.... A more recent count has placed the number of existing techniques well over 400."[24] While it has not yet reached the point where there are as many brands of therapy as there are therapists, there is certainly a variety of approaches for a therapist to use. Such diversity creates choices for people who are seeking help. The situation, however, may be confusing.

Let me try to clarify this situation. First, it is important to recognize that most therapies have some elements in common. For example, most therapists provide a supportive atmosphere for the patient: they are interested in the patient and his or her well being. Also, the relationship that develops between therapist and patient is important in almost all therapies. Moreover, almost all therapies have an effect on the restoration of morale. The patients usually experience a regeneration of hope. They become more enabled and energized and can begin to do things for themselves, which has the effect of rebuilding confidence.

Second, you will find that many therapists are not doctrinaire. They take an eclectic position, picking out what seems to work best for their patients from what is available in the different therapeutic techniques. Moreover, many therapists continue their education after graduate or professional school, learning new, innovative techniques.

It may be helpful to briefly describe some of the major approaches to therapy that are being used to treat depression. Three of the better-known approaches are (1) *psychodynamic therapy*, in which the focus is on intrapsychic conflicts, (2) *cognitive-behavioral therapy*, which focuses on thought processes and behavior and (3) *interpersonal therapy*, which focuses on human relationships.

Psychotherapy as we know it began with Freud and his invention of psychoanalysis. Psychoanalysis is both a complex theory about human personality and a technique for treating emotional disorders, particularly those disorders that have been labeled as neuroses or neurotic behavior. Therapies that draw heavily on Freud's psychoanalytic theories are usually referred to as psychodynamic therapies.

Psychodynamic therapies focus on conflicts within the person. Typically these conflicts have their roots in childhood experiences, and

[24]*Kazdin (1986), p. 96.*

often in parent-child relationships. The roots of these conflicts are not usually accessible to the patient. Much of the troubling material is believed to be out of the patient's awareness, or in Freud's term, *unconscious*. In order to resolve the conflicts that underlie the patient's current symptoms, it is important in psychoanalytic therapies to bring this material into the open. The analyst works with the patient to bring these ideas to light and shows the patient how they relate to her or his current problems.

In classical psychoanalysis, making what is unconscious known is accomplished by such techniques as free association and dream analysis. In free association, the patient speaks about whatever is on her or his mind, trying not to hold back anything or to suppress any idea. The patient's flow of ideas tends to form links with unconscious materials. In dream analysis, free association is used to work back from the dream content to the unconscious materials that are believed to have given shape to the dream. In the procedure, the patient is asked to freely associate to different parts of the dream. During therapy, the analyst tries to stay in the background and allow the patient to talk. She or he listens attentively, trying to pick up clues about the conflicts that are causing distress in the patient. From time to time the analyst will interpret the patient's narrative, linking current materials to events of the past, offering some explanation of what has happened in the patient's life.

One of the important ideas in psychodynamic therapies is the concept of transference. Transference is a replay or revival, in a current relationship, of conflicts that remain unresolved from earlier experiences, particularly those involving parent-child relationships. A basic tenet of psychodynamic therapy is that the feelings and thoughts of these prior relationships arise again in therapy, with the therapist finding himself or herself in a position very much like the parent. Feelings of love, anger or dependency that develop toward the therapist are part of this transference. Transference is felt to be an essential part of therapy, but the process should be resolved by the time therapy is terminated.

Freud's approach to therapy was originally developed to deal with such emotional disorders as hysteria and obsessive-compulsive behaviors. He later turned his attention to depression in *Mourning and Melancholia*, pointing to the experience of loss and internalized anger as important aspects of the problem. Over the years a number of writers in the psychoanalytic movement have expanded on Freud's thinking about depression. These writers include Karl Abraham, Otto Fenichel, Edith

Jacobson and Leopold Bellak.[25] Bellak presented a rather comprehensive list of the issues he believed psychoanalytic therapists should pay particular attention to in treating depression. The list includes problems relating to self-esteem, a severe super-ego, aggression turned against the self, feelings of loss, feelings of disappointment, feelings of having been deceived by others, dependence on positive input from other people, an excessive need to be loved and use of denial as a defense mechanism.

Bellak's list suggests the kinds of issues one might anticipate being addressed in a contemporary psychoanalytic approach to depression. These problems are clearly important, but could take considerable time to cover in therapy, particularly in psychoanalytic therapy, which traditionally proceeds at a slow pace. However, Bellack believes that if the therapist is sensitized to these issues, effective therapy for depression can be carried out in a relatively short period of time. Typically, the therapist will approach these issues by exploring the life history of the patient, considering recent incidents that triggered the depression, and pointing out common denominators between the past and present to improve the patient's understanding and insight.

Other psychodynamically oriented therapists interested in the possibility of radically shortening the course of treatment but still drawing on the legacy of Freud's ideas have developed various forms of *brief dynamic therapies*. In these therapies, the therapist does not try to deal with all of the patient's personality problems; rather, the therapist and patient focus on an important problem area. They attempt to deal with this problem in a limited number of sessions, usually less than 20.

Within these restrictions, the therapist will view symptoms from a psychoanalytic or modified psychoanalytic framework and use some of the techniques of psychoanalysis. The therapist may analyze defense mechanisms, show how current symptoms have their roots in early childhood experiences, and interpret relationships in terms of transference.

In contrast to traditional psychodynamic therapy, which delves deep into the personality and may take years to complete, cognitive therapy is usually carried out in a matter of weeks or months. The basic premise underlying cognitive therapy is that depressed emotion is triggered in large part by maladaptive thought patterns. The objectives of cognitive therapy are to work with the patient to identify maladaptive thought

[25]*See Bellak (1981) for a discussion of psychoanalytic thinking about depression.*

patterns and then to help the patient change these patterns—to begin to think in ways that are adaptive rather than disabling. In his book *Cognitive Therapy and the Emotional Disorders,* Aaron Beck spoke of the challenge to psychotherapy as one of giving the patient effective techniques to overcome his or her faulty perceptions. The therapist reaches the patient's emotions through the patient's cognitions. Beck proposes that by correcting faulty beliefs, the excessive, emotional reactions will be diminished.[26]

We have previously discussed some of the typical maladaptive thought patterns found in patients experiencing depression, including perfectionist and black-and-white thinking. The patient may not be aware of these tendencies, and if he is, may not see anything wrong in thinking this way. He may not see that these patterns are causing trouble. The therapist attempts to discover these thoughts and help the patient understand their role in the depressive problem.

In the early stages of cognitive therapy, the therapist tries to elicit from the patient any automatic thoughts that the patient has been experiencing. Later, the therapist will attempt to weave these fragmented thoughts into more general patterns—the views that the person has about him- or herself, his or her life and the outside world. As an aid in therapy, the therapist may ask the patient to keep a diary to record thoughts that occur during feelings of depression. The therapist will discuss the material in the diary during the therapy hour.

In cognitive therapy, the therapist might ask questions like "Before you started feeling sad this morning, what were you thinking about? What was on your mind?" Or, "When you were lying awake last night and couldn't get to sleep, imagine you had a tape recorder, recording your thoughts. Try playing some of that tape back for me. What would it sound like?" The questions may vary, but the objective is to bring out the patient's thoughts, particularly those automatic thoughts that are believed to trigger and sustain depressed mood.

To illustrate a cognitive therapy approach, here are some excerpts from a case reported by Jeremy Safran and his colleagues. The client, a 25-year-old male, was being treated for depression, apathy and pro-

---

[26]*Beck (1976), pp. 213–14. Robert DeRubeis and his colleagues (1990) suggest that the basis for the effectiveness of cognitive therapy lies not only in the changes in thinking that take place in therapy, but in the active application of their principles in the patient's everyday life. The same maxim would seem to hold for most forms of therapy; therapy does not stop in the therapist's office. One must practice what one has learned.*

crastination. At the time of entering therapy he had been thinking about applying for admission to a university, but found himself unable to get moving. During the stage of therapy illustrated here, the therapist was concerned with uncovering the thought processes that were supporting this pattern of immobilization.

The client told the therapist that he planned to have his transcripts sent to the university; instead, he found himself lying in bed, thinking of telephoning the transcript office but not doing so. The therapist asked the client to recall how he was feeling at the time and to relate any images or thoughts that seemed relevant. The young man described how he imagined the people in the transcript office would react to his call. "I see a picture of some of the people that I have to contact to try to get something moving on this and I see them hating me. They see me as a nuisance." He imagined that he would receive a curt, unpleasant response, something like, "Sorry you've got your answer and that's all there is to it." On afterthought, he added that this fear was probably ridiculous.

The therapist commented that the fear was real for the client. The client agreed that it was indeed very real. As the session continued, the therapist asked him to elaborate on his imagery. "Like I'm lying here in bed and the thought occurs to me 'this is what I've got to do. I've got to phone this woman.' Ah . . . it's funny, after describing all this, suddenly it doesn't seem as surprising to me, that what happens is that I stay in bed for another hour."

The client later observed, "Yeah. I can see when I was lying there in bed thinking . . . 'I should call the transcript office,' the other part of me was saying 'No way . . . I'm not going to call that woman.'" The therapist asked whether he could make a case for not calling the woman. The client replied, "You bet I can!" He then related automatic thoughts, catastrophizing the scenario. He saw the woman as threatening and himself as powerless and helpless. "And suddenly, it's like I'm wrong and she's in the right. I can imagine her saying 'I'm going to call the principal,' and it's like I've got to hang up and run and hide."

The therapist observed that it was like he was a powerless child who had done something wrong. The client agreed, "Yeah, I'm in the wrong. And I'm gonna get squashed like a bug. And I have no defense, no defense at all."[27]

---

[27]*Safran et al. (1986). The case study is related on pages 516–18.*

The interchange had elicited a group of automatic thoughts suggesting a self-image of a powerless child victimized by powerful and threatening adults. As therapy continued, other tendencies of the client—to seek the approval of others and not to express his own anger became clearer in light of this fundamental perception of powerlessness and his exaggerated fear of retaliation. In later sessions, the therapist was able to work along with the young man to take a more critical look at these debilitating ideas and successfully challenge them.

One of the techniques of cognitive therapy is to challenge the maladaptive beliefs—the basic assumptions of the patient that are believed to underlie the depression. An effort is made to break through the patient's closed systems of thought, to open up the patient's thinking so that he or she can entertain new information and alternative ways of looking at problems. The process of challenging the patient's beliefs is not unlike a Socratic dialogue and sometimes can have the flavor of a debate. The therapist may bring up facts and counter examples that tend to question and contradict the negative mind sets of the patient. At times, the actions of a cognitive therapist resemble those of a lawyer for the defense of the patient, and particularly his or her self-esteem.

Like brief dynamic and cognitive therapies, interpersonal psychotherapy (IPT) is designed to be time limited and can be carried out in a few months. IPT provides an alternative focus to the treatment of depression, moving away from the patient's psyche and belief systems to his or her interpersonal relationships. Since we know that interpersonal stresses often trigger the onset of a depressive episode, it makes sense to consider these problems in treating depression. IPT endeavors to help the patient develop more effective ways of coping with the interpersonal problems that appear to have played a role in bringing on the depression.

The therapist tries to identify the interpersonal problems that are of central importance to the patient; then the therapist helps the patient deal more effectively with the problems. The IPT therapist is particularly sensitized to look for problems in four areas: grief, interpersonal disputes, changes in roles and interpersonal deficits such as loneliness.

With regard to grief, the therapist looks for indications of abnormal grief—reactions to loss that have not been resolved in a reasonable period of time. The therapist tries to help the patient facilitate the mourning process and free him- or herself from a crippling attachment to someone who has gone.

With regard to interpersonal disputes, the therapist looks for possible problems with the patient's spouse, children, other family members, co-workers and friends. If significant disputes are uncovered, the therapist and the patient will try to work out plans to better resolve the disputes. The plans might involve changing the patient's expectations about the people involved or trying to improve communication with the other people.

There are many role changes or transitions that may be associated with the onset of depression. Think of such changes as leaving for college, getting married, becoming a parent and changing jobs. As indicated earlier, such changes often generate stress, and high levels of stress can trigger depression. The therapist looks for difficulties that have occurred during these role transitions. As the therapist explores these changes, he or she looks for losses of familiar support in the patient's life, how the patient has managed emotions such as anxiety or anger that have been aroused by the transition and whether the patient has experienced loss of self-esteem. The therapist also assesses the types of new social skills that may be required to cope effectively with the changed situation. The therapist tries to help the patient put the old role in perspective, as well as to acquire the skills needed in the new role.

With regard to loneliness and social isolation, we know that loneliness and depression are highly related. In helping the patient cope with this problem, the therapist explores the patient's past and present relationships and employs techniques such as *role playing* to diagnose specific difficulties the patient may have in communicating and relating to others.

Role playing is a technique in which the therapist and patient engage in a spontaneous drama. The therapist and patient each take a part (role) in a situation in which they make up their lines as they go along. For example, let's say that therapist Debra Carter is working with a patient, Don, who has great difficulty asking a woman for a date. Dr. Carter may play the part of the woman Don is interested in. She and Don will engage in a dialogue in which he asks her out. Dr. Carter may critique Don's performance, helping him to sharpen his approach. Practice in role playing may improve Don's skill and confidence.

In the book *Interpersonal Psychotherapy of Depression,* the developers of this technique provide case examples illustrating the way IPT is carried out. One example would be the case of Ellen F, a woman whose central problem involved role transition.[28] Ellen had been in an

[28]*Klerman et al. (1984).*

unhappy marriage for about ten years. She had married at age 17, in part as a way of escaping an overintrusive mother. Her husband turned out to be an alcoholic who when intoxicated could be both verbally and physically abusive. Ellen had an abortive affair, which proved disastrous, precipitating her suicide attempt. Ellen wanted to end the marriage but found herself incapable of doing so. She hoped therapy would help her take this step.

After beginning therapy she asked her husband to leave the house; he proved more than willing to do so, having complaints of his own. Therapy then focused on helping Ellen manage the transition out of marriage. The therapist helped her identify new social relationships to fill the vacuum left by the shattered marriage, helped her deal with her fears of being alone, and helped her understand that her own self-worth should not depend on having a man to call her own.

Therapy also strengthened her resolve not to reconcile with her husband when he came back and asked her to try again. She realized that being lonely for a period of time was better than the misery that she had been through.

During therapy, Ellen widened her circle of friends and began dating again. When therapy ended she had not reached the point where she had achieved a comfortable life, but she had made a difficult transition away from a destructive situation.

Effectiveness of Therapy

How effective is psychotherapy in the treatment of depression? Are some approaches to therapy more effective than others in the treatment? Does the competence of the therapist make a difference in the outcome of therapy? Are there characteristics of the patient that make a difference in whether therapy will be effective? These are some of the questions that researchers have posed and are seeking to answer in clinical studies. These questions are important both to the practitioner of therapy and to the person in need of therapy.

In conducting research to answer these questions, investigators must exercise considerable care in the way they design and carry out their studies to ensure that their results are as clear-cut as possible. For example, in studying the effectiveness of therapy, researchers are careful to ensure the following:

1. All patients included in the study are clearly diagnosed as depressed. The selection of patients is often based upon both a clinical interview and psychological testing.
2. The patients selected for inclusion in the study are randomly divided into two groups: one group receives therapy, the other group is put on a waiting list for treatment and serves as a control group.
3. Measures of evaluation are taken before therapy begins, at the end of therapy and at a subsequent follow-up time. The evaluations often assess various symptoms of depression to permit the researchers to determine in which areas therapy is most effective.

Many carefully designed studies have now been carried out comparing patients given psychotherapy with patients serving as controls. The results are clear. Most patients given psychotherapy are helped by the treatment. Patients who complete psychotherapy are usually less depressed than control subjects who are not given therapy. As is true for antidepressant medications, some patients are not helped by psychotherapy.

While there is ample evidence that psychotherapy is effective in the treatment of depression, there still remains some question as to *how* effective. When a person is improved, what precisely do we mean? Do people who are treated by psychotherapy achieve the same level of well being as people who were not depressed to begin with? The answer is probably no. While improved, people who are treated for depression are still likely to experience higher levels of depressive symptoms than "normal" people.[29]

To use a very rough analogy, therapy for depression in some respects is like treatment for chronic diseases such as heart disease or arthritis. Treatment for such conditions helps control symptoms and prevent flare-ups of the problems. Likewise, in psychotherapy for these diseases, one may not find a magic bullet that cures the problem of depression like an antibiotic wipes out a bacterial infection. After psychotherapy, the person prone to depression usually feels a lot better and should be in a better position to effectively manage him- or herself, which will reduce the chances of further symptoms. But underlying genetic vulnerabilities remain and the problems in the environment that triggered the depression may also remain. There is a clear potential for further problems.

[29]See Nietzel et al. (1987).

Having shown that psychotherapy is effective in the treatment of depression, researchers turned to the question of comparing different types of therapies. Is one approach to therapy for depression more effective than another? This is a very practical question for anyone considering therapy; one would like to know which approach is most likely to be beneficial.

In "comparative outcome" studies, patients are randomly assigned to one of the several types of treatments under investigation. Particular care has to be given so that all types of therapy are carried out in the clinical trials in the manner in which they are designed to be carried out. Evaluation measures usually include psychological testing and clinical interviews.

To date, the tentative conclusion from comparative outcome studies is that there is not much difference between the therapeutic approaches tested in terms of their effectiveness in treating depression.[30] There are some practical consequences of this observation. People looking for help can pay attention to the qualities of the individual therapist and how they relate to the person without worrying too much about the technical aspects of therapy. Also, prospective patients can select an approach that is short term and feel some confidence that they will be helped. There is little evidence at this point to indicate that a person is likely to profit more by undergoing long-term, deep therapy to deal with an ongoing depressive problem. A person may want to choose long-term, intensive therapy for other, more fundamental reasons, but it is not usually necessary for the alleviation of depressive episodes. If proponents of long-term, intensive therapy could demonstrate that the effects of such therapy are more robust—that there is less chance of a recurrence of depressive symptoms—a stronger case could be made that it is the treatment of choice for depression.

Let's talk about the individual therapist. Doctors, lawyers and teachers differ in how competent they are and this can make a difference in what you get from them. A good lawyer may win your case for you, a bad one may lose it. In much the same way, a skilled therapist is more likely to do more useful things in therapy than a less skilled therapist. Observations of ongoing therapy indicate that a skilled therapist is more

---

[30]*There are a number of studies that show little difference in the effectiveness of different types of psychotherapy in the treatment of depression. An example is Gallagher & Thompson (1982).*

likely to help patients explore issues and problems and to do so without arousing the patient's hostility or causing unnecessary distress. Researchers have reported a relation between the competence of the therapist and the extent to which a patient improves during treatment for depression.[31]

As the skill of a therapist can make a difference in the outcome of therapy, the question that must inevitably arise is how does one find a good therapist? This is not an easy question to answer, but here are some ideas. Probably the most useful benchmark in choosing a therapist is how effective he or she has been with previous patients. Unfortunately, this kind of information is unlikely to be available in a systematic way. No one takes polls of this situation. However, it is possible to ask around. If someone has been to a therapist, you should be able to find out whether the person felt the therapist was helpful and what the therapist was like as a person. People who have been to a therapist are an important source of information about her or him.

If you cannot get a likely name from a friend, then your next best bet may be the referral services of the local professional associations for psychiatrists, psychologists and clinical social workers. The referral services will usually give you several names of people who are licensed practitioners. They may also have background information about each person, which will allow you to make some inquiries. If you decide to call one of the names, see if you can talk briefly with the therapist on the phone to gain a sense of what he or she is like and whether you feel comfortable talking with the person. You should also ask about fees. If they are way out of line, you might want to try someone else. A sky-high fee does not guarantee a better therapist, it only guarantees a poorer pocketbook.

Some other possible sources of referral are community mental health associations and the psychology, psychiatry and social work departments of local universities. You will also find listings of these professionals in the Yellow Pages of your phone book.

Let's now turn our spotlight away from the therapist and onto the patient. Are there characteristics of patients that may make a difference in whether therapy is likely to prove helpful? Certainly one of the most important factors is how depressed the patient is when he or she enters therapy. People who begin therapy feeling mildly or moderately depressed

[31]*See O'Malley et al. (1988).*

are more likely to emerge from therapy in decent shape than people who are severely depressed.[32] Individuals whose personal and social resources are in better condition to begin with are likely to do well.[33]

Another factor is the patient's attitude. If the patient has a positive attitude about psychotherapy—that it can help—the chances are better that it will help. This "expectation factor" is not only important in psychotherapy, it plays a role in almost all kinds of human healing processes. Hope and belief are important in the treatment of physical problems as well as emotional problems.

Hospitalization for Depression

When should a person be hospitalized for the treatment of depression? As a general rule, hospitalization should be considered when the patient's symptoms are unmanageable through outpatient care. Two clearcut cases of this are when the depression includes psychotic features such as delusions and when the patient is overtly suicidal.

Many depressed people think about suicide; some talk about it. When a person is openly suicidal, there may be little choice but to consider hospitalization. It may be impossible to adequately monitor the person's behavior and protect her or him against self-harm outside of a hospital setting.

Psychiatric hospitals can provide care and safety for the severely depressed patient. Throughout the United States there are both public and private psychiatric hospitals. The National Institute of Mental Health has compiled lists of these hospitals, as well as outpatient clinics. In addition, you can probably obtain information about hospitals in your area by calling your state mental health agency.[34] Judging from the brochures that inundate private practitioners, some of the private psychiatric hospitals look very attractive, resembling resorts more than the infamous asylums of the not-too-distant past.

Psychiatric hospitals may offer several modalities of treatment for depressed patients. These include medication, individual and group therapy and electroconvulsive shock treatment. With regard to therapy,

[32]See, for example, Gonzales et al. (1985), and Hoberman et al. (1988).
[33]See, for example, Hoberman et al. (1988).
[34]See Warsack et al. (1985).

you may find increased emphasis on group therapy in hospitals. The patients are all gathered together under one roof, which can reduce or eliminate scheduling problems. In addition, group therapy is cost-effective for a hospital; one therapist can work with a number of patients simultaneously. Group therapy can be of particular benefit to patients whose problems have to do with difficulties in interpersonal relations. One learns to relate by relating and group therapy provides a relatively safe training forum in which to learn.

Electroconvulsive therapy is referred to in scientific journals as ECT, and has been popularly called "shock treatment." Electroconvulsive therapy has been described as "the most controversial treatment in psychiatry." The author of that statement is no less than a prestigious panel of psychiatrists, neurologists and other scholars marshaled by the National Institutes of Health (NIH) to evaluate the use of ECT in the treatment of mental and emotional disorders.[35]

Electroconvulsive therapy has been used as a psychiatric treatment for over 50 years. During that time it has earned a fearsome and sometimes unsavory reputation. Fearsome because the procedure of a patient being rendered unconscious, given electric shocks and going into convulsions is a scary idea, and in its early use often produced serious harmful effects on patients. Unsavory because in some institutions, ECT was used as a means of controlling the behavior of difficult, unruly patients.

The bulletin issued by the NIH panel tells us that in the early days of ECT use, there was a relatively high mortality rate—about one death per thousand patients. As many as 40 percent of the patients experienced major problems, the most common being vertebral compression fractures.[36]

Fortunately, the safety of the procedure has been dramatically improved. Death and serious medical complications are now rare. The procedure, however, is not benign; there are still some risks involved and there are often undesirable effects.

Following is a description of electroconvulsive therapy drawn from the statement issued by the NIH panel. ECT is administered in the early morning after a period of fasting of from eight to twelve hours. An anticholinergic agent is given before treatment. An intravenous line is placed

[35]*Consensus Development Conference Statement (1985), section 5, conclusion.*
[36]*Consensus Development Conference Statement (1985), section 2.*

in a peripheral vein of the patient and an anesthetic is given, which is followed by a muscle relaxant. This permits the patient to sleep through the ECT procedure and reduces convulsions. Electrodes are placed on the patient's head and then a small electric current is administered. The idea is to administer the smallest amount of electric energy necessary to induce a seizure. Seizures are monitored by an electroencephalogram, which measures brain wave activity, or by other procedures.

During the first minutes following electric shock, the patient's cardiovascular system is disturbed. There may be transient changes in pulse and blood pressure and cardiac arrhythmias. The patient's cardiac response is monitored closely during the procedure.

When the patient awakes after ECT, he or she is often confused. There may be temporary memory loss and headaches. Sometimes it takes several hours for the patient to regain clear consciousness. The larger the electric shock and the more frequently the procedure is carried out, the more severe this confusional state is likely to be. The patient's ability to learn and remember can be adversely affected for several weeks after ECT. Some patients complain that their memory was impaired for a much longer time. Some patients related to the NIH panel that ECT was a terrifying experience.

With all of these negatives, why use ECT? Indeed, many people take a dim view of it. In some institutions the use of ECT has been curtailed. In some areas it isn't used at all. The rationale for ECT, however, is that it can be an effective treatment for certain kinds of depression that may not respond to more conservative treatments. ECT may be particularly useful in treating patients whose depression includes psychotic symptoms such as delusions. It can also be useful for severely depressed patients who do not respond to medications or psychotherapy, and for patients who are overtly suicidal.

Evaluation studies indicate that ECT seems to be at least as effective as antidepressant medication on hospitalized patients. In one study, patients given ECT had shorter hospital stays than patients given antidepressant medications.[37]

These studies indicate that for patients with severe depressive problems that are unresponsive to medication and therapy, ECT is an option to consider. The patient should be fully informed about the procedure and his or her consent obtained.

[37]*See Markowitz et al. (1987).*

Relapse and Recurrence

Follow-up studies of patients who have been treated for unipolar depression indicate that the longer range effects of treatment are variable. There are great individual differences. The good news is that some people do very well. In a study carried out in California following up with patients who had been treated in hospitals and community mental health centers, Andrew Billings and Rudolf Moos found that many patients were not only experiencing few depressive symptoms, but had improved self-esteem and were coping better with stressful events. And although they still had relatively few friends and the interactions within their families were not as supportive as they could be, their social lives were getting better.

In contrast to these ex-patients who are doing quite well, we know that many other patients experience a recurrence of depressive symptoms. The bad news is that neither treatment by medication or psychotherapy is a guarantee that a person who has recovered substantially from an episode of depression will remain symptom free. And the same holds true for persons who have received ECT. According to published reports, the chances are approximately one in three that a person treated for unipolar depression will experience a recurrence of depression within a year or so. The odds rise to about one in two after two years.[38]

The risks of recurrence of depression seem greater if (1) the depression treated was severe, (2) there is a high genetic predisposition for depression as evidenced by the presence of depression in other family members, (3) the person continues to show evidence of neuroendocrine dysregulation on such tests as the DST, (4) the person continues to live in an environment that engenders a great deal of stress and (5) the person receives weak support from family and friends.[39] If the person has a history of intermittent depression, the risk of further episodes is obvious. Untreated bipolar depression has a high risk of recurrence.

I previously mentioned some of the things that people can do to help themselves in preventing episodes of depression. The question arises, "Is there a role for professional help in the prevention of recurrence of depression?" The panel of experts convened by the National Institutes

---

[38]*See, for example, Gonzales et al. (1985).*

[39]*See Belsher & Costello (1988) for a critical review of factors relating to relapse of unipolar depression.*

of Health to evaluate the use of antidepressant medications stated their belief that antidepressive drugs may have value as a prophylaxis against the recurrence of depression. The panel indicated that this is particularly true for the use of lithium as a preventive measure in bipolar depression. The panel stated, "Lithium is the drug of choice for preventing recurrence of bipolar depression." In keeping patients on lithium maintenance, the panel advised physicians "to maintain the patient on the lowest dose that prevents the return of symptoms since these lower concentrations are associated with fewer side effects."[40]

Although the panel acknowledged that research on the use of tricyclics for preventing the recurrence of unipolar depression was not yet sufficient, the panel nonetheless suggested the use of tricyclics for this purpose. The panel suggested using dose levels for these drugs similar to or somewhat lower than the doses used during the acute phase of the depressive episode.

With regard to the use of psychotherapy as a preventive measure, it would take some rethinking of the traditional model of psychotherapy to utilize therapy as a preventive technique. In the traditional mode of therapy, a patient comes to the therapist with problems, has these problems thoroughly aired and hopefully resolved, and is then discharged. This traditional approach is based on an implicit assumption that bringing up and working through unresolved conflicts will result in a "cure" for the patient. While this may or may not be so for most emotional problems, we know that depression has a high rate of recurrence, so a different type of model may be more appropriate in treating depression. This model postulates that for many patients, there is a need for continuing contact on a much-reduced level between therapist and patient after initial discharge. It may be something like coming in for a visit once or twice a year—or, more importantly, when things begin to get rough.

My view is that for people who have suffered from recurrent depression, the time to see your psychotherapist is when stress is building up. Why wait until the stress level passes your tolerance level and the chances of a severe depressive reaction loom large? Wouldn't it be better to consult the therapist with whom you previously worked to help you over the difficulties *before* things get out of hand? This is the view I leave with my patients when they have finished the primary course of therapy.

[40]*Consensus Development Conference Statement (1984), sections 4 and 5.*

A position along these lines was advanced by a research team at the University of Oregon. Having completed a follow-up study of people with unipolar depression who were treated by cognitive-behavioral approaches, researcher Linda Gonzales and her colleagues wrote, "The results suggest that although most patients are improved at the end of treatment, for some this improvement is relatively transient and by the LIFE criteria does not constitute recovery from the episode that led them to seek treatment. A potential implication of these results for cognitive-behavioral treatments is that they are either too short to produce more enduring improvement in a greater proportion of patients and/or that they need to be supplemented with posttreatment maintenance and booster sessions to assist patients in maintaining the improvements they make in treatment."[41] And indeed, a study carried out by I. M. Blackburn and his colleagues found that a group of patients who continued to work with therapists after their initial symptoms had abated were less likely to experience relapses into depression.

BIBLIOGRAPHY

Beck, A. T. (1976). *Cognitive therapy and the emotional disorders.* New York: International University Press.

Bellak, L. (1981). Brief psychodynamic psychotherapy of nonpsychotic depression. *American Journal of Psychotherapy,* 35, 160–72.

Belsher, G., & Costello, C. G. (1988). Relapse after recovery from unipolar depression: A critical review. *Psychological Bulletin,* 104, 84–96.

Billings, A. G., & Moos, R. H. (1984). Treatment experiences of adults with unipolar depression: The influence of patient and life context factors. *Journal of Consulting and Clinical Psychology,* 52, 119–31.

_____, & _____ (1985). Psychosocial processes of remission in unipolar depression: Comparing depressed patients with matched community controls. *Journal of Consulting and Clinical Psychology,* 53, 314–25.

Blackburn, I. M.; Eunson, K. M.; & Bishop, S. (1986). A two-year naturalistic follow-up of depressed patients treated with cognitive therapy, pharmacotherapy and a combination of both. *Journal of Affective Disorders,* 10, 67–75.

Consensus Development Conference statement (1984). Mood disorders: Pharmacologic prevention of recurrences, 5, no. 4. National Institutes of Health.

_____ (1985). *Electroconvulsive therapy.* 5, no. 11. National Institutes of Health.

[41]*Gonzales et al. (1985), p. 467.*

Conte, H. R.; Plutchik, R.; Wild, K. V.; & Karasu, T. B. (1986). Combined psychotherapy and pharmacotherapy for depression. *Archives of General Psychiatry*, 43, 471–79.

Davidson, J. R. T.; Giller, E. L.; Zisook, S.; & Overall, J. E. (1988). An efficacy study of isocarboxazid and placebo in depression, and its relationship to depressive nosology. *Archives of General Psychiatry*, 45, 120–27.

DeRubeis, R. J.; Evans, M. D.; Hollon, S. D.; Garvey, M. J.; Grove, W. M.; & Tuason, V. B. (1990). How does cognitive therapy work? Cognitive change and symptom change in cognitive therapy and pharmacotherapy for depression. *Journal of Consulting and Clinical Psychology*, 58, 862–69.

Dobson, K. S. (1989). A meta-analysis of the efficacy of cognitive therapy for depression. *Journal of Consulting and Clinical Psychology*, 57, 414–19.

Elkin, I.; Shea, T.; Watkins, J. T.; Imber, S. D.; Sotsky, S. M.; Collins, J. F.; Glass, D. R.; Pilkonia, P. A.; Leber, W. R.; Docherty, J. P.; Fiester, S. J.; & Parloff, M. B. (1989). National Institute of Mental Health Treatment of Depression Collaborative Research Program: General effectiveness of treatments. *Archives of General Psychiatry*, 46, 971–82.

Folkenberg, J. (1983, October). Using drugs to life that dark veil of depression. *FDA Consumer*. HHS publication no. (FDA) 84–3140.

Freud, S. (1959). *Mourning and melancholia*. In *Collected Papers*, vol. 4, 152–70. New York: Basic Books.

――――― (1963). *Therapy and technique*. New York: Collier.

Gallagher, D., & Thompson, L. W. (1982). Differential effectiveness of psychotherapies for the treatment of major depressive disorder in older adult patients. *Psychotherapy: Theory, Research, and Practice*, 19, 482–90.

Georgotas, A., & McCue, R. E. (1986). Benefits and limitations of major pharmacological treatment for depression. *American Journal of Psychotherapy*, 40, 370–76.

Gonzales, L. R.; Lewinsohn, P. M.; & Clarke, G. N. (1985). Longitudinal follow-up of unipolar depressives: An investigation of predictors of relapse. *Journal of Consulting and Clinical Psychology*, 53, 461–69.

Hoberman, H. M.; Lewinsohn, P. M., & Tilson, M. (1988). Group treatment of depression: Individual predictors of outcome. *Journal of Consulting and Clinical Psychology*, 56, 393–98.

Hollon, S. D.; Shelton, R. C.; & Loosen, P. T. (1991). Cognitive therapy and pharmacotherapy, for depression. *Journal of Consulting and Clinical Psychology*, 59, 88–99.

Hough, R. L.; Landsverk, J. A.; Karno, M.; Burnam, A.; Timbers, D. M.; Escobar, J. I.; & Regier, D. A. (1987). Utilization of health and mental health services by Los Angeles Mexican Americans and non–Hispanic Whites. *Archives of General Psychiatry*, 44, 702–9.

Jamison, K. R., & Akiskal, H. S. (1983). Medication compliance in patients with bipolar disorder. *Psychiatric Clinics of North America*, 6, 175–92.

――――――; Gerner, R. H.; & Goodwin, F. K. (1979). Patient and physician attitudes toward lithium: Relationship to compliance. *Archives of General Psychiatry*, 36, 866–69.

Kathol, R. G., & Henn, F. A. (1983). Tricyclics – The most common agent used in potentially lethal overdoses. *Journal of Nervous and Mental Disease*, 171, 250–52.

Kazdin, A. E. (1986). Comparative outcome studies of psychotherapy: Methodological issues and strategies. *Journal of Consulting and Clinical Psychology*, 54, 95–105.

Klerman, G. L.; Weissman, M. M.; Rounsvaille, B. J.; & Chevron, E. S. (1984). *Interpersonal psychotherapy of depression*. New York: Basic Books.

Knesper, D. J.; Wheeler, J. R. C.; & Pagnucco, D. J. (1984). Mental health service providers' distribution across counties in the United States. *American Psychologist*, 39, 1424–34.

Kocsis, J. H.; Frances, A. J.; Voss, C.; Mann, J. J.; Mason, B. J.; & Sweeney, J. (1988). Imipramine treatment for chronic depression. *Archives of General Psychiatry*, 45, 253–57.

Markowitz, J.; Brown, R.; Sweeney, J.; & Mann, J. J. (1987). Reduced length and cost of hospital stay for major depression in patients treated with ECT. *American Journal of Psychiatry*, 144, 1025–29.

Nietzel, M. T.; Russell, R. L.; Hemmings, K. A.; & Gretter, M. L. (1987). Clinical significance of psychotherapy for unipolar depression: A meta-analytic approach to social comparison. *Journal of Consulting and Clinical Psychology*, 55, 156–61.

O'Malley, S. S.; Foley, S. H.; Rounsaville, B. J.; Watkins, J. T.; Sotsky, S. M.; Imber, S. D.; & Elkin, I. (1988). Therapist competence and patient outcome in interpersonal psychotherapy of depression. *Journal of Consulting and Clinical Psychology*, 56, 496–501.

Prien, R. F. (1981). *Information on lithium*. DHHS publication no. (ADM) 81-1078. National Institute of Mental Health.

_____, & Gelenberg, A. J. (1989). Alternatives to lithium for preventive treatment of bipolar disorder. *American Journal of Psychiatry*, 146, 840–48.

Prozac: Fluoxetine hydrochloride. (1990). *Comprehensive Monograph*. Dista: Eli Lilly and Company.

Rancurello, M. (1986). Antidepressants in children: Indications, benefits, and limitations. *American Journal of Psychotherapy*, 40, 377–92.

Rapp, S. R.; Parisi, S. A.; Walsh, D. A.; & Wallace, C. E. (1988) . Detecting depression in elderly medical inpatients. *Journal of Consulting and Clinical Psychology*, 56, 509–13.

Regier, D. A.; Goldberg, I. D.; Taube, C. A. (1978). The de facto U.S. mental health services system: A public health perspective. *Archives of General Psychiatry*, 35, 685–93.

Sackeim, H. A. (1985, June). The case for ECT. *Psychology Today*, 19, 36–40.

Safran, J. D.; Vallis, T. M.; Segal, Z. V.; & Shaw, B. F. (1986). Assessment of core cognitive processes in cognitive therapy. *Cognitive Therapy and Research*, 10, 509–26.

Sargent, M. (1986). *Depressive disorders: Treatments bring new hope*. DHHS publication no. (ADM) 86-1491.

Shaw, E. D.; Stokes, P. E.; Mann, J. J.; & Manevitz, A. Z. A. (1987). Effects of lithium carbonate on the memory and motor speed of bipolar outpatients. *Journal of Abnormal Psychology*, 96, 64–69.

Small, I. F.; Milstein, V.; Miller, M. J.; Malloy, F. W.; & Small, J. G. (1986). Electroconvulsive treatment—Indications, benefits, and limitations. *American Journal of Psychotherapy*, 40, 343–56.

Steinbrueck, S. M.; Maxwell, S. E.; & Howard, G. S. (1983). A meta-analysis of psychotherapy and drug therapy in the treatment of unipolar depression with adults. *Journal of Consulting and Clinical Psychology*, 51, 856–63.

Taube, C. A.; Burns, B. J.; & Kessler, L. (1984). Patients of psychiatrists and psychologists in office-based practice: 1980. *American Psychologist*, 39, 1435–47.

Teicher, M. H.; Glod, C.; & Cole, J. O. (1990). Emergence of intense suicidal preoccupation during fluoxetine treatment. *American Journal of Psychiatry*, 147, 207–10.

Ursano, R. J., & Hales, R. E. (1986). A review of brief individual psychotherapies. *American Journal of Psychiatry*, 143, 1507–17.

Warsack, M. R.; Henderson, P. R.; Witkin, M. J.; & Manderschild, R. W. (1985). *Mental health directory*. DHHS publication no. (ADM) 85-1375. National Institute of Mental Health.

Weissman, M. M.; Meyers, J. K.; & Thompson, W. D. (1981). Depression and its treatment in a U.S. urban community—1975–1976. *Archives of General Psychiatry*, 38, 417–21.

Yokopenic, P. A.; Clark, V. A.; & Aneshensel, C. S. (1983). Depression, problem recognition, and professional consultation. *Journal of Nervous and Mental Disease*, 171, 15–23.

Conclusion

Depression, like other mental and emotional disorders, is a worldwide problem. One is likely to find the disorder in every corner of the globe. Joseph Westermeyer put it this way: "Psychiatric signs and symptoms are remarkably consistent from culture to culture. Patients everywhere complain of insomnia, worry, crying spells, . . . weakness, . . . suicidal ideation."[1]

Depression is not a new problem that has arisen in the wake of our modern technologically advanced society, although we may well be witnessing an increase in its prevalence. Judging from historical sources, it seems likely that depressed mood and depression have plagued humankind from time immemorial. The ancient Greeks were well aware of these problems and one can find stories in the Bible that portray some very depressed people. Think of the prolonged malaise that afflicted King Saul, and of young David trying to soothe his moods with music.[2]

While depression has been a problem for a long time, until recently we have not had much understanding of it or known how to treat it effectively. There were a few spots of light in this void. Freud, for example, offered some theoretical contributions highlighting the role of loss in depression and suggesting that self-directed anger plays a role in the disorder. Descriptive psychiatry produced some categories for classifying types of depression, but the distinctions were not all that clear and the terms were not universally accepted. In their early investigations, the biologically oriented researchers found little to write home about and the attention of research psychologists was turned elsewhere to problems that were more amenable to study.

[1] *Westermeyer (1987), p. 475.*
[2] *The Bible describes how King Saul was tormented by an evil spirit from the Lord and how David played his lyre, which refreshed Saul, and the evil spirit departed. I Sam. 16: 14–23.*

Over the past few decades the situation has changed dramatically. Psychological and psychiatric journals have become inundated with research on depression. Researchers have been hard at work both improving the techniques needed to better study depression and producing substantive knowledge about the causes of depression and its treatment.

In listing the advances in knowledge brought about by this flurry of activity, one could begin by pointing to better methods of diagnosing depression. This has resulted in part from more clarity about the symptoms of depression. The *Diagnostic and Statistical Manual,* for example, lays out specific criteria to help the researcher and practitioner in making diagnoses. In addition, we now have psychological measures that can indicate with reasonable accuracy the presence of depression in adults. These measures are not only useful in the clinic, they can also be used for large-scale studies in the community.

Community surveys have revealed that all groups in our society are susceptible to depression. Racial or ethnic background doesn't seem to make a great deal of difference in whether a person is at risk for depression. Gender and age are probably better indicators of risk. For reasons that we can only speculate about, women seem to be more vulnerable than men. And people in the prime time of life, those who have major responsibility for carrying out the workload of the society, seem to be at greatest risk. The latter finding points to stress as one of the factors that trigger depression. And, indeed, many psychological studies support this idea. Changes in life, particularly those involving personal loss, are related to depression. Cumulative stresses whether major or minor may also bring on depression.

Still, we know that not everyone subjected to stress becomes depressed. Studies have shown that the way we appraise stressful situations makes a difference. If we don't exaggerate the importance of what is happening, we are less likely to overact and less likely to experience an emotional downswing.

The way we think about things makes a difference. Both theory and research indicate that thought patterns such as overgeneralization, perfectionist and absolutist thinking and a predilection for fixing blame on oneself can interfere with making a rational appraisal of a stress-provoking situation. Instead of reacting in a measured, problem-solving way, the tendency is to overreact, catastrophizing the situation, opening up the floodgates to depression.

While psychological researchers have been unraveling the thought processes that trigger and sustain depressed mood, researchers trained in the biological sciences have been exploiting new technologies to study the relation of depressed mood and the functioning of the body. Significant discoveries have been made linking depressed states to aberrations in the neurotransmitters in the brain. Genetic links to depression are being explored, particularly for bipolar disorder. The day may not be far off when biological tests will be used in the diagnosis and treatment of depression.

The discoveries of the last decades have greatly increased our understanding of depression and raised hope and expectations for better things to come. We should anticipate both fuller understanding of the depressive process and improved techniques of treatment.

Today the mental health profession can offer antidepressive medicines and psychotherapy. Both treatments are usually effective. The medicines may improve mood and get a person functioning. Therapy can help change maladaptive thought patterns and destructive patterns of living. While both types of treatment are helpful, neither is a panacea. Medicines have side effects that may not be tolerated by some patients. Therapy takes time and is expensive, and the patient has to be willing to put in the required time and effort. A minority of patients are not helped by either medication or therapy.

Perhaps the biggest problem with current treatments for depression is that once the course of treatment is completed, there is a sizeable risk that in time—perhaps even in a matter of months—the symptoms may reappear. Not everyone experiences recurrence of symptoms, but enough people do to make it a worrisome possibility. At this point in time we are not certain of the best ways to prevent recurrence of depressive episodes. For bipolar disorder, the consensus is that using lithium as a prophylaxis may be helpful in eliminating or reducing the severity of mood swings. There may also be value in the continued use of medicines for unipolar depression after the initial episode has abated. I have recommended that when patients begin to experience uncomfortable levels of stress in their lives, this is the time to consult their therapists, not wait until everything falls apart. A stitch in time may well save nine.

There is a good deal patients can do for themselves to help prevent further episodes of depression. A life-style that reduces the risk of depression is within the power of many people, just as a life-style that reduces the risk of a heart attack. In the latter case, if you stop smoking, keep your weight down, avoid dietary fats and unneeded salt and engage in a prudent program of exercise, the chances of developing coronary heart disease drop considerably. To reduce the risk of depression, you have to pay attention to the build-up of stress in order to take actions that keep it within acceptable limits. You should aim for a balanced life-style that includes activities that are personally gratifying.

It is also important to look at what is happening in life from a perspective that does not turn everyday problems into overwhelming ones. Give yourself a break when things go wrong. Don't get down on yourself to the point you can't make a comeback tomorrow. Remember that everyone has bad days. The trick is to learn to take them in stride. Research tells us that people who don't catastrophize events are less likely to become depressed.

In this book I have tried to present information and ideas that may be helpful to people who have experienced some of the symptoms of depression or have seen such symptoms in others who are close to them. I hope that this information will be useful in increasing your understanding of the nature of depressed mood and depression and the options that are available in dealing with these problems.

I have tried to emphasize prevention and the importance of healthy attitudes and a balanced life-style. But when depressed feelings are severe or one has been in the throes of a protracted malaise that has eroded the joy of life, one would do well to consider consultation with a mental health professional. This book was not intended as a substitute for such consultation. I hope, however, that it will assist you in making an informed decision about what to do if such a time should come to pass.

Index

181